"This is a hard book to read—like watching the news and learning about war, poverty, and famine. We would rather look away, ignore, and pretend. God doesn't pretend; he knows, he enters in, and he loves us. And God calls us to participate in his love and presence. So for those with family or friends walking through the confusion and challenges of dementia, this book is a real gift. Groothuis takes us from admissions of moments of rage to the sweet, tender mercy of Sunny the goldendoodle, from painful, honest reflections about the eeriness of the disease to signs of hope that only God can provide. He helps us begin to understand what is beyond our grasp. Many who try to make sense of their own journeys will find here an authentic voice to help along the way."

Kelly M. Kapic, professor of theological studies, Covenant College, author of *Embodied Hope*

"To be honest, I've never read a book like this. It overflows with deep reflection on the suffering of life and the apparent absence of God at the very times we need him most. But the specialness of this book lies in Groothuis's raw, unfiltered, and bewildering expression of emotion— pain, agony, confusion—regarding the journey of his dear wife, Becky, and its impact on Doug's own pilgrimage. There are no cheap Christian slogans, no slapping of a Bible verse as a Band-Aid on a near-mortal wound, no simplistic happily-ever-after. But there is hope. Hope built on deep reflection about Christianity, suffering, and the meaning of life. To me, this is the best book my dear friend has ever written. Its healing powers will penetrate your soul as you slowly read through its pages."

J. P. Moreland, distinguished professor of philosophy, Talbot School of Theology, Biola University

"Poignant. Profound. Powerful. This very personal journey through a wife's dementia will astound you with its eloquence and insights. The path through twilight is painful, but—thank God!—it's not without ultimate hope. This is a memoir that will mark you forever."

Lee Strobel, professor of Christian thought, Houston Baptist University, author of *The Case for Christ* and *The Case for Faith*

"Douglas Groothuis's *Walking Through Twilight* is an extraordinarily moving memoir of lament. In inviting the reader into the experience of his wife's progressive dementia, he combines superb writing and the incisive thinking of a first-rate philosopher, which he is. But far beyond this, the book is filled with liberating honesty and the particular beauty of unadorned truth. Hearing God in the thunder and lightning is easy, but hearing him in what sounds mostly like silence takes a particularly keen and delicate ear, one this author possesses in abundance."

Eric Metaxas, radio host of the Eric Metaxas Show, author of *Bonhoeffer: Pastor, Martyr, Prophet, Spy*

"Would I write as Doug Groothuis does here? Could I even begin to? I was profoundly humbled by this memoir. Philosophers are all about clear thinking, but the classroom is beggared by the anguish described here with such searing honesty, such poetic insight, such intense clarity, and such unconquerable hope."

Os Guinness, author of *Impossible People*

WALKING

THROUGH

TWILIGHT

A WIFE'S ILLNESS—
A PHILOSOPHER'S LAMENT

DOUGLAS GROOTHUIS

FOREWORD BY NICHOLAS WOLTERSTORFF

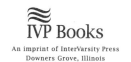

IVP Books

An imprint of InterVarsity Press
Downers Grove, Illinois

InterVarsity Press
P.O. Box 1400, Downers Grove, IL 60515-1426
ivpress.com
email@ivpress.com

InterVarsity Press® is the book-publishing division of InterVarsity Christian Fellowship/USA®, a movement of students and faculty active on campus at hundreds of universities, colleges, and schools of nursing in the United States of America, and a member movement of the International Fellowship of Evangelical Students. For information about local and regional activities, visit intervarsity.org.

All Scripture quotations, unless otherwise indicated, are taken from The Holy Bible, New International Version®, NIV®. Copyright © 1973, 1978, 1984, 2011 by Biblica, Inc.™ Used by permission of Zondervan. All rights reserved worldwide. www.zondervan.com The "NIV" and "New International Version" are trademarks registered in the United States Patent and Trademark Office by Biblica, Inc.™

While any stories in this book are true, some names and identifying information may have been changed to protect the privacy of individuals.

Chapter 6, "Learning to Lament," is adapted from Doug Groothuis, "Learning to Lament," Journal for Baptist Theology & Ministry 10, no. 2 (fall 2013), 70-73. Used by permission.

Chapter 17, "My Escape into Meaning," is adapted from Douglas Groothuis, "Bedeviled by My Wife's Dementia," Christianity Today, October 26, 2015. Used by permission.

Photo of Becky and Sunny courtesy of John Mervill.
Cover design: Cindy Kiple
Interior design: Daniel van Loon
Images: dramatic sunset: © Ilona Wellmann / Trevillion Images
        twilight landscape: © bjorn 999 / iStockphoto / Getty Images

ISBN 978-0-8308-4518-7 (print)
ISBN 978-0-8308-8900-6 (digital)

Printed in the United States of America ♾

InterVarsity Press is committed to ecological stewardship and to the conservation of natural resources in all our operations. This book was printed using sustainably sourced paper.

Library of Congress Cataloging-in-Publication Data
A catalog record for this book is available from the Library of Congress.

P	25	24	23	22	21	20	19	18	17	16	15	14	13	12	11	10	9	8	7	6	5	4	3	2	1
Y	36	35	34	33	32	31	30	29	28	27	26	25	24	23	22	21	20	19	18	17					

Bitter-sweet

Ah, my dear angry Lord,
Since thou dost love, yet strike;
Cast down, yet help afford;
Sure I will do the like.
I will complain, yet praise;
I will bewail, approve;
And all my sour-sweet days
I will lament and love.

GEORGE HERBERT

CONTENTS

Foreword

NICHOLAS WOLTERSTORFF

BECKY, THE WIFE OF THE AUTHOR of this volume, was extraordinarily gifted with words. The gift began to fail her. She was diagnosed as suffering from primary progressive aphasia, a form of dementia that has, as one of its primary signs of mental deterioration, the inability of the person to find words to say what she wants to say. *Walking Through Twilight* is the author's lament for the wide and deep losses that this ravaging disease has wreaked in his life and that of his wife. He does not wallow in the horror of the disease, but neither does he gloss over it or look away. He does not flinch from the painful reality.

Walking Through Twilight is more, however, than an unfailingly honest lament over loss. Interspersed with Groothuis's lament is a series of meditations, evoked by observing the nature and course of the disease, and his response and that of others, whose aim is to understand something of the hand of God in this valley of suffering and to discern how to live lovingly and faithfully in this shadowy place.

Groothuis is a philosopher and theologian, steeped in Scripture. So the meditations are, as one would expect, philosophical and theological in their overall character, and rich—incredibly rich—in their incorporation of passages from Scripture, especially from the wisdom literature of the Old Testament. But the meditations are never abstract. In each instance they are tied to the author's observation of his wife's suffering, and his response and that of others. The image that comes to mind is that of a cord on which beads are strung—beads of reflection strung on a cord of lament over loss.

And what an astute observer Groothuis is! Soon after his wife's diagnosis became known, he noticed that people began to speak differently to her. They would "raise their voice," "lapse into singsong and upward inflection, and refer to her in terms they would never use for any right-minded adult—terms like *hon* or *dear* or other inapt terms of awkward endearment." In short, they would speak to her condescendingly. That observation leads Groothuis into a lovely meditation on what is wrong with speaking condescendingly to such a person—or, indeed, to any person—and how to speak to such a person instead.

Another example: he notes that he still laughs and wonders whether, in this sea of loss, it's appropriate for him to laugh. And he observes that his wife also still laughs, though what she laughs at has changed significantly. She no longer laughs at jokes; she doesn't get the point. The meditation closes with these poignant words: "Proverbs lauds the wise and hard-working woman. 'She can laugh at the days to come' (Proverbs 31:25). Becky cannot laugh at the days to come, but in these days—or at least some of them—laughter will come to both of us."

One more example: the author found himself getting intensely angry at the way in which some members of the medical profession treated Becky, especially at the way in which she was treated in a "behavioral health unit"—and at the way he was treated. This leads him into a probing meditation on the role of anger in life. He also finds himself getting angry with God. And *this* leads him to reflect on whether it is right, sometimes, for a Christian to be angry with God. Does anger at God have a place in the Christian life?

These examples illustrate the point that the author does not stop with lament over loss but over and again looks ahead by reflecting on how to live well amidst this loss. The title and subtitle say it all: a philosopher's lament over his wife's illness intertwined with reflections on how to walk through this twilight. The examples also illustrate another distinctive feature of the book: the specific and the general are seamlessly interwoven. Observation of the specific evokes reflection, reflection illuminates the specific.

Introduction

WALKING
THROUGH TWILIGHT

Hope deferred makes the heart sick,
but a longing fulfilled is a tree of life.

PROVERBS 13:12

SINCE I WAS RELEASED from graduate school, no one has told me
what to write. After my doctoral committee accepted my dissertation in 1993, I have written books, articles, editorials, reviews, and
letters to the editor. Perhaps I am spoiled, but I work hard at my
writing. Writing for me is not *therapeutic.* I have never written
merely to make money or *express myself* (a common curse inflicted
by egotists on readers). I have been reluctant to write a memoir. The
task of extending the knowledge of God, defending "the faith that
was once for all entrusted to God's holy people" (Jude 3), and ap-
plying the Christian worldview to the whole of life has been my
passion, however flawed my efforts. But perhaps I can combine
memoir, lament, and philosophical reflection.

Most of my work responds to attacks on Christianity or to
corruptions within it. Becky was there near the beginning. We met

in 1983 when we worked for a campus ministry. As we got to know each other and fell in love, she encouraged two things that changed my life for the better. First, she convinced me that the time was over for research and that I should begin writing my first book. Second, she offered to edit the chapters as I went along. That book, *Unmasking the New Age*, is my bestselling book. We were and are united in our sense of calling. Becky edited all my books, except *Philosophy in Seven Sentences* and this offering. That is one of my reasons for lament.

This book is different from all my others. I did not want to write it, but it wanted to be written. Publishers and friends urged me to write it, but I tried to turn them down. However, I found that not writing the book would be harder than writing it. Unlike my other books, it is not strictly linear or expositional. Unlike *Christian Apologetics*, for example, it is not one long argument for Christianity. *Walking Through Twilight* is only autobiographical for the sake of being pastoral, philosophical, and theological. Expressing myself is not the point, but I need to recount my experiences—some of them raw, many of them tragic—to offer courage, hope, and meaning amidst the distinctive suffering of dementia care. But how much should I write about myself? A pastor and long-time friend recently told me that my previous book *Philosophy in Seven Sentences* was his favorite of all my books. (I did not ask how many of them he had read.) His reason surprised me. He said it was because I revealed more of myself in that book. I did, but this book enters new territory for me as a writer. It is a *memoir*, heaven help us. But as I enter my seventh decade on earth and my fifth decade as a Christian, I hope my reflections are worth beholding. I agree with Bertrand Russell that "a long retrospect gives weight and substance to experiences."[1]

I call this book *Walking Through Twilight*. I chose *twilight* instead of *darkness* since I wrote this book while Becky is at home and I can still communicate with her. When this changes, it will be *darkness*, and I won't write of that. However, Becky and I know that the darkness of the crucifixion is followed by the light of the resurrection. She will be raised immortal in God's good time. Dawn follows darkness, but this comes at the price of agonized waiting. This book is a witness to that waiting.

A memoir contains autobiography, but is not an autobiography proper. Memoir recounts part of one's life that the author takes to be worth sharing with the wider world. It is a difficult genre to do well. And this is my first attempt. At least I will give you many biblical passages and quotations from many wise authors.

Oddly, a memoir should not be self-centered. Rather, the self should be centered in a place fit for noting and conveying needful truth to others. Since we are made in God's image and likeness, and since Christians are taught and directed by the Holy Spirit (at least when we are not quenching or grieving him), our lives can be worth a memoir. I hope my reflections on the dark drama of dementia will set up a few guideposts and illuminate a few dark places. We can walk through twilight and into the night with courage, and hope for a new dawn at the far side of suffering.

While reflecting on two paintings of Christ, the poet W. H. Auden wrote that suffering is often hidden from a world not suffering at that moment.[2] While human and beast go about their business, some of us are suffering the "dreadful martyrdom" of being a dementia caregiver. The pedestrian and the agonized soul who walk side by side; perhaps one can learn from the other.

Of course, dementia gets worse, but this memoir is not written as a strict chronology. Rather, I explore themes related to episodes in the devolution of Becky. Writing of "the progression of her disease" is too tame and bloodless. The phrase hints at some manner of *progress*. But there is no progress, no advance. I must let the words fall and root where they should.

Some of my chapters, such as "Learning to Lament," are longer and more philosophical than the rest. I encourage readers to press on through those chapters, nevertheless, since they give a richer meaning to the others and explain the reason for the hope I have (1 Peter 3:15). My strategy concerning chapters is to give a taste of what my lament is and then to explain how we may cope with such laments. This is followed by more chapters explaining the vicissitudes and exigencies of Becky's and my journey.

I often interrupt or augment my narrative with observations that, on occasion, become excurses. These are not rabbit trails but reflections on this darkening footpath. I am a philosopher, and it is philosophy that often saves me from malignant melancholy.

Becky gave me permission to write this book. I told her that writing it was helpful to me and might assist others going through similar ordeals. I put things in perspective by saying to her, "All your work as a writer, editor, and speaker came out of *your strength*. Now this book can encourage people through your *weakness*." She weakly smiled and chuckled a bit, the way people do when they hear something insightful, but a bit ironic. Becky will not edit this book, nor will she read it, but she has authorized it, and I dedicate it to her.

One

RAGE IN A PSYCH WARD

How can we sing the songs of the
LORD while in a foreign land?

PSALM 137:4

THE YEAR OF 2014 SAW MY WIFE spend five weeks in the hospital
to diagnose mental problems. When she came back, we had to
revise how we lived and how we saw the future. It was miserable. It
was the worst year of my life, as it was for Becky. I learned a raft
of things I never wanted to know. This chapter recounts learning
to adjust to having my wife in a psychiatric unit.

Before Becky went into the hospital, she and I saw a neurologist
for one year who was sure Becky did not have dementia. He was
wrong, because he was only thinking of Alzheimer's disease. But
Becky has a rare form of dementia, called primary progressive
aphasia (PPA). Every time I say those three words, it hurts.

My year of learning began with the protocols of a psychiatric unit.
After Becky and I and a friend spent twelve hours in the emergency
room, the psychiatrist finally arrived and put Becky on a seventy-
two-hour hold in a behavioral health unit in a hospital across town.
I saw her hauled out on a stretcher with almost no belongings. I had

never seen her more pathetic, but she did not complain, probably because she was not aware of her surroundings. When I questioned the men about what possessions she should have, one said, "She won't need many of her belongings there." I had no idea what he meant until I entered the unit the next day.

I left the hospital with my loyal friend, drove home, greeted my upset and lonely dog, and then listened to Pink Floyd's *Dark Side of the Moon*. My dog, Sunny, lay not far from me. Somehow this was what I had to do. This renowned classic rock recording reminds me of Ecclesiastes, but without God. That was how I felt.

The next day, after many calls to doctors, my friend Sarah and I visited Becky in a behavioral health unit across town. Unexpectedly, we had to pass through a security check and leave keys and wallets outside before the door was unlocked to let us in. What kind of place was this? Entering the patient area, I saw Becky wandering around in tears. No one was attending to her. We locked eyes and embraced. She pointed me to her room and we went in to talk. A nurse quickly scolded us, saying that I could not share the room (even with the door open) with my wife of thirty years. I was shocked and angry, but complied. I drew up several chairs in the open area.

My friend and I sat down to talk to Becky in this most inhospitable hospital. We were disturbed by a young man talking loudly on a pay phone. I asked him to not speak so loudly. He rebuked me. I yelled at him to shut up. The anger and confusion within me was turning into rage second by second. I wanted to kill him, so great was my rage. Of this, I am ashamed. A nurse pointed her finger at me and shouted at me to shut up. My friend and I were banished to a meeting room outside the open area.

I was so angry and irrational that I began to blame my friend for Becky's psychiatric incarceration. We were kicked out. It was entirely my fault. I later realized that I might have been arrested had I not left when commanded to. That would look good for my school, "Christian Philosopher Arrested for Causing a Riot at a Psychiatric Ward." It was a near miss.

This episode and several others began to show me the futility of rage. Paul was right to warn that rage is not from the Holy Spirit but of our fallen human nature. He places rage in unholy company:

> The acts of the flesh are obvious: sexual immorality, impurity and debauchery; idolatry and witchcraft; hatred, discord, jealousy, fits of rage, selfish ambition, dissensions, factions and envy; drunkenness, orgies, and the like. I warn you, as I did before, that those who live like this will not inherit the kingdom of God. (Galatians 5:19-21)

In "How the Soul Discharges Its Emotions Against False Objects When Lacking Real Ones," the essayist Montaigne instructed me that the actions of rage—stomping, screaming, and throwing things—do nothing to rectify the enraging condition. We merely "beat at the air" or "beat our breasts."[1] When applied, this wisdom helps contain rage and cuts off the escalation into destructive actions. At bottom, though, advice, no matter how sagacious, cannot substitute for the work of the Holy Spirit. Opposed to the "acts of the flesh" are "the fruit of the Spirit."

> But the fruit of the Spirit is love, joy, peace, forbearance, kindness, goodness, faithfulness, gentleness and self-control. Against such things there is no law. Those who belong to Christ Jesus have crucified the flesh with its passions and desires. (Galatians 5:22-24)

I returned to the hospital the next morning and apologized to everyone I could. Becky was peacefully eating breakfast next to a kind woman. She was soon transferred to another behavioral health unit. There too I found myself confused and sometimes infuriated by their rules and the authority they had over my own wife and me. I shouted at innocent people who were only following rules.

Whenever I left Senior Behavioral Health, the doors locked behind me. Some try to escape. I don't blame them.

After several visits and more apologies, I learned the protocol of this sad but necessary place. Over five weeks I visited Becky nearly every day. The drive to and from was about sixty miles, so visiting, while still teaching, was taxing. God met me in these visits. I had been re-reading Viktor Frankl's classic study of suffering and meaning, *Man's Search for Meaning*. Human value can be affirmed in the thick of searing suffering, as he found in Hitler's prison camps. But we have to change ourselves. "When we are no longer able to change a situation . . . we are challenged to change ourselves."[2]

I could not magically free Becky—or any of the other sad patients—from this necessary but sorrowful place. However, I could smelt meaning out of suffering. I could not deny the suffering of confusion, fear, and loneliness, but I could live within it without dying from it. Again, Frankl says,

> We who lived in concentration camps can remember the men who walked through the huts comforting others, giving away their last piece of bread. They may have been few in number, but they offer sufficient proof that everything can be taken from a man but one thing: the last of the human freedoms—to choose one's attitude in any given set of circumstances, to choose one's own way.[3]

Becky was my first concern in behavioral health. I would usually visit during meals, and encouraged Becky to eat. She ate little (and emerged from the hospital five weeks later nearly emaciated). At dinner, Becky would often fall silent and hang her head. I would try to comfort her, but also was alert to the predicaments of the other patients. I would greet them, talk, offer to pray for them, and in some cases pray with them.

I became familiar with some of the patients, especially those who stayed more than a few days. There was Cindy, always shaking and paranoid. She asked me, "If I pray out loud, will Satan hear my prayer and hurt me?" I assured her that God was greater than Satan and that she should not worry about that. She was reassured.

There was Jack, a tall, friendly man, who was depressed. I heard him say, "I love to sleep. I would sleep my life away if I could"—a classic symptom of intense depression. I have tasted of it, but have not been poisoned. Jack was also a hypochondriac, pestering the nurses to check his symptoms. There was so much to pray for.

Another woman was, I think, schizophrenic. I started to talk with her, but she quickly grew angry and had a verbal tantrum about God knows what. Then this poor soul looked at my wife. Their eyes met and locked, and they both smiled wordlessly. Strange love visited the psychiatric ward through my wife. This was common, I was told.

Becky, often wordless and ever confused, ignited joy in distressed people. Once when I was visiting for dinner, a woman introduced my wife as "our movie star," referring to her good looks. There is love in the ruins, if one has eyes to see.

When my friend and I picked up Becky from behavioral health, a nurse and several others cried over her departure. She could not sign the release papers, so I did. I have learned to take over many of Becky's responsibilities. I am her advocate and mediator. These are Christlike roles, but I am far from sinless.

Two

THE YEAR OF LEARNING THINGS I DID NOT WANT TO KNOW

When we came into our home from the five-week hospital stay, our dog, Sunny, literally leaped for joy. He had missed Becky badly. Even now, two-and-a-half years later, he still runs to Becky when we have been away. He gets around to me later. Sunny's joy was the happiest thing about returning. What followed was not.

We soon discovered that home would not be our old home; it often seemed more like a prison. After a few weeks of agonized futility, I decided we needed a live-in caregiver.

I learned how to accommodate another person living in our home to help Becky. God provided someone quickly. But we did not adjust quickly. Neither did our caregiver, despite her experience in serving sick people. Becky was no longer the *woman of the house* (to use an antiquated phrase). She had to cede some control to a stranger. I was the reluctant referee in these squabbles; no one else could be. I got to know Lana and tried to sympathize with her disappointing life. We got on for about nine months, and then she burned out.

Our next caregiver was mellow, quiet, and less high-strung than our previous helper. But she only stayed about six months. She left because she was preparing for marriage. Further, she could not provide the level of care Becky needed. In one sense, no one could.

Through this, I have become an employer. Given my gift of disorganization, this is a daunting but necessary area of my learning. Much of my life after Becky's diagnosis has been *daunting but necessary*. I am pressed into service by exasperating conditions beyond my control. Most of us are, eventually.

After her hospitalization, I was told by a psychiatrist to become her guardian and conservator. As guardian, I can make all the legal and medical decisions. As conservator, I am in control of her finances. Conservatorship is an ordeal involving many calls, emails, and trips to my lawyer. The lawyer's work is not *pro bono*. Nor am I their best client. I learned how to set up guardianship and conservatorship for my wife, which gives me legal and financial authority. Becky used to attend to all our financial concerns. She did so with precision and promptness. I simply gave all of it over to her—checks, bills, and notices—with perfect confidence. Then, even before her diagnosis, she lost her ability to add up sums. She gave it all back to me, the organizationally adolescent one. (If God ever gave me the gift of administration, it would be akin to him raising the dead.)

I learned what it felt like to stand in front of a judge with our lawyer and my wife to hear him say, in effect, that I was now her parent. On the way home from this ordeal, Becky melodramatically said, "You own me." I don't blame her. I had never used my role as a husband to contradict her wishes—well, I did a few times, in the first few years of marriage. Now she was my charge, and we both hated it. Our relationship would continue to change under the tyranny of her disease.

After Becky returned I tried to learn how to "play hurt" (in the sports sense) to a greater degree than ever. In the weeks and months after Becky's hospitalization, I had to cancel some speaking engagements. One of my three classes was taken over by another professor. However, I debated an atheist in Boulder during the first week of Becky's hospital stay during that time. I continued writing, which is my life's calling. God has always empowered me to teach, preach, and write. I would sometimes walk into the classroom without adequate notes, feeling desperate and undone, yet still engage a class in my areas of expertise. This was a sprout of grace in a field of sorrow. I could soldier on—earthbound, not on eagles' wings.

I learned depths of sorrow and distress I had never known before. Years ago, a colleague spoke to me of his wife's tribulation with cancer. She had said to him, "I did not know the human body could bear so much pain." I never forgot that. Little did I know how much psychological agony a human soul could bear. Yet my suffering could not be compared with the suffering of Jesus Christ, my Savior. When he cried out, "My God, my God, why have you forsaken me?" he experienced suffering of the highest possible degree (Matthew 27:46). He was an innocent victim, "the Lamb of God, who takes away the sin of the world" (John 1:29). God was now making me an expert in suffering. I wish he had picked someone else. But as a philosopher I must ponder the meaning of suffering, as I am attempting to do in this little book, the one I never wanted to write.

I researched the possibility of long-term assistance for Becky. After my insurance provider told me they covered it, I found that my insurance did not cover it. Much of this crucible is not covered by anything, it seems. But I still know (in my better moments) that

> Whoever dwells in the shelter of the Most High
>> will rest in the shadow of the Almighty.
> I will say of the LORD, "He is my refuge and my fortress,
>> my God, in whom I trust." (Psalm 91:1-2)

Becky memorized all of Psalm 91 when she went through an earlier crucible of an anomalous staph infection. She would recite it on the way to the infectious disease doctor. She can no longer recite this psalm from memory or memorize anything new. Yes, God has all of this trial covered, but this divine covering (for us) did not keep suffering at bay. No, this covering is a way *through suffering*, not a way to *escape suffering*.

I tried to learn how to verbally communicate with my once-brilliant wife in ways she could understand. Since she is declining, I have to attempt to relearn this often, and I often fail. I can complete some of her sentences, but not all. Eventually, there will be no sentences at all. That day may not be far away.

I learned how it feels to weep often and to cry unexpectedly, even in public. When my eyeglasses are smudged, and I take them off to look at them, I often find the marks of tears. I now behold much of the world through tears and am alert to the tears of others. I also cry inside without tears, because tears and the paroxysms that often accompany them get in the way of doing what I must do. God must count those uncried tears too. David, my brother in lament, wrote,

> Record my misery;
>> list my tears on your scroll—
>> are they not in your record? (Psalm 56:8)

I also learned things that were not miserable.

I learned that so many friends helped or offered to help, including good people at Denver Seminary, where I work. This includes meals brought over, help with moving one helper out and moving another in, help with legal and financial problems, and much more.

I learned that God brings good out of even the most horrible suffering. This year was a crucible, excruciating. This word *excruciating* means to take on a cross. It was invented as a reflection on the passion of Jesus. If we take the cross of Christ, we can become a bit more like Christ, more aware of others' suffering, and more willing to listen and help.

I learned that I can keep praying when I am not happy with God. I once believed that prayer was reserved for certain emotional states. To be joyful or thankful is to be prized, but God is still there when those emotions escape us. I take heart in the many psalms of lament.

This was my miserable year of learning things I did not want to know. It was the worst ever. But then I recall that at one time 2008 was the most miserable year of all. As were 2009, 2010, 2011, 2012, and 2013. And so I go on.

Three

THINGS FALL APART

Things fall apart; the centre cannot hold;
Mere anarchy is loosed upon the world.
WILLIAM BUTLER YEATS, "THE SECOND COMING"

WHEN ORDINARY TASKS of communication become complex, then difficult, and then impossible, isolation becomes inevitable. Helping becomes excruciating. Consider the telephone—not smartphones but the simple landline telephones—which we usually do not. Nothing is simple or normal to one suffering from dementia. I have used the phone without difficulty for over fifty years. The phone for me is not the phone for Becky. Things fall apart. She is alienated from simple technology because her brain has rendered even the simplest tasks daunting, if not unmanageable.

Becky did not have a telephone in her bedroom for some time, since she cannot now initiate calls or receive many. However, I sometimes want to call her without having our caregiver mediate the connection. And I cannot expect the caregiver to come back to work when she is off-duty. Becky's best friend, Sharon, wanted to call Becky to encourage and pray for her. So, with little optimism, we installed a landline in her bedroom. (There is no hope for Becky using a cell phone.) I believe our success rate was zero. I often called home to hear only the ringer and no voice. Unless our caregiver is home to help, Becky is a stranger to all things telephonic—exiled from a commonplace. Little is common anymore; more is alien now. Consider an example.

Becky walked down to my study with the portable landline phone in her hand. Looking puzzled and desperate (her typical expression now), she stammered out that she could not understand it. Words failed her and me, since I could not orally explain the simple device. I said, "Let's pretend I am calling you and that my table is the base. Ring, ring. Now you pick it up." She picked up the remote control for my stereo instead. "No, pick up the phone," I said, pointing to it. She picked it up and held it to her ear upside down. "You need to put it right side up." She did. "Now push the button to answer it." That instruction, like many others, was just a cluster of human noises to Becky. I took the phone—amazingly, not getting angry—and showed her the chosen button. Her eyes saw the phone, her limbs could perform the request, but her brain could link neither words nor my despairing gestures to the meaning *push this button to hear a voice.*

"Just put the phone upstairs where you found it and we will worry about it later." (I now try to placate Becky by deferring failures to an indefinite future when we will address them again. But I seldom do, having been defeated by the ordinary recurrently.) She went upstairs. As I began to read a new book, *How to Listen to Jazz*, I heard the soft footsteps again. She then appeared from around the corner of books. Then I saw the signature hand gestures and heard the belabored words of my aphasia-stricken wife. Given a few words I could associate with recent events, I realized that she probably had not put the phone back on its base properly. I confirmed this by picking up the landline extension next to me.

My patience broke a bit as I sighed and lumbered from the basement to the second floor. (I labor more at this, given the onerous weight that dementia places on my soul and body, and Denver's mile-high altitude.) Becky followed me up. At the first floor, I asked, "Did you leave it in your room or is it somewhere else?" Predictably, she did not know. I trudged upstairs, entered Becky's gloomy room, and found the phone on its base, but placed bottom up. Instead of resting in the base, it perched upon it—something I had not seen before. Oddly, it seemed almost regal in its absurdity. The phone was displaying its simple hardware for the world to see, more like a statue on its base than a phone orphaned of its home. I put it where it belonged and realized that this phone would serve only as an unused ornament, testifying to further futility and isolation. Becky is isolated, unkindly removed, from friends who could call her. Besides the technology, she is isolated from me and me from her. We cannot have a simple conversation about an everyday object. Things fall apart.

The telephonic heartbreak just narrated took about ten minutes. I marvel at how many mistakes it contained. One of them, taken by itself, might be humorous, as when we absentmindedly botch a simple action. (I know. I am a philosophy professor.) These miscues clustered in only a short time, but time slowed down. The compacting of deep mistakes—each odd, unlikely, and taken together almost eerie—made the episode *extraordinary* in its unnerving heartbreak. Extraordinary is usually used to commend a person, event, argument, or object as *better than the ordinary*. I use it to mean *below the ordinary* in a remarkable way. The odds are against this many mistakes being made this quickly and with such heartbreak. The event stands out to me. Becky and I will experience more of these episodes until the very undertaking of simple tasks will not enter her mind.

Things fall apart. The mind miscarries. Telephones fail. Communication wilts and dies. Isolation ensues. "Mere anarchy" is not loosed upon *the world*, as Yeats wrote, but *near anarchy* is loosed upon one hapless married couple, who are feeling their way through the darkness. Yet our center does hold.

Interlude

THE MENSA CARD

ONLY TWO MONTHS AFTER Becky and I moved into our present home, she was put into Senior Behavioral Health at Lutheran Medical Center. The move had been hectic and deeply disordering. We had lived in our old home for twenty years. It was stuffed and difficult to move, especially the 140 boxes of books. My students and friends did most of the book work. But even as I write three years after we moved, many things are out of place.

There is a desk in Becky's bedroom. But it is no longer used as one. Pens, pencils, staplers, notes, and so on are no longer part of her world. The desk supports a small stereo system. Recently, I pulled out one of the drawers to find what I could use at my desk. I found a key to our lockbox, which I thought was lost. Sadly, it was too late. I had already had the old lock drilled open and replaced.

I uncovered a number of out-of-date business cards, Becky's old driver's license, her Arizona State ID card, and . . . her Mensa membership card. Of course, I remembered that she was in this "International High IQ Society" in the early to mid-nineties. I persuaded her to join, since it would add to her prestige as a budding writer and speaker. Mensa only takes members who have a certifiably genius IQ. While I am skeptical of IQ as the best way to consider intelligence, it hit the mark for Becky. She joined, but not much came of it. She had kept the card, which was "valid through 3/31/94."

She let it lapse not long after, since she did not see much value in membership, but saw not a little self-congratulation in the group.

At first, after finding the card, I mentally put it in the capacious category of *things not pertaining to Becky anymore*. But it stood out as a poignant marker of loss, an exhibit from such different days. I would not throw it out. I wept as I held it and thought about it. She was so brilliant. I loved that about her. Now that is gone, but she is not. And she knows—for now—what she has lost.

I don't have a Mensa card and never will. I often told people that Becky was more intelligent than I am. She was. She signed the card *Rebecca M. Groothuis* in her impeccable cursive handwriting. Today, she cannot write a word. She cannot read. She might remember Mensa, but I am not going to bring it up.

Four

IT IS EERIE

I did not expect it to be eerie. Dementia is many things, none pleasant, most maddening, and all taxing on the ones suffering and on their caregivers. Strangely, I find that *eerie* is sometimes the right word for the odd and mystifying unraveling of a human being.

Dementia is not only a loss. It is a shift from normality to abnormality, from health to sickness, from integration to disintegration. Dementia negates the right workings of the brain, taking away and reordering what is left. But it is not the order of a well-curated exhibit of paintings or the order of a lecture well-given or the order of a pitch well-delivered in baseball. *Order* is, in fact, the wrong word—although it comes to mind readily. There is a new arrangement of parts and systems in the brain; the demented brain, corrupted and decaying, tries to right itself while it sinks.

Disorder is the word to use—and we mourn its use. But this disorder fits into patterns, which are at least partially recognizable. Those with aphasia are at a loss for words. I am too, on occasion, but the words usually come when summoned ("It will come to me"), although as I age, they are sometimes late in arriving. If they refuse my summons, a conversation partner may rope them in for me. Those with aphasia can think an idea and never divine the word on their own.

My wife needs help to find words, particularly nouns. Oddly, she often says in perfect English with no hesitation, "I can't talk anymore." (I sometimes tell her this is a self-refuting statement, and she often gets it.) She repeatedly says a few agitated words, makes gestures, and hopes I can rescue her from the anguished and quaking silence. This becomes a pattern of pathos. That is, a pitiful arrangement congeals out of malfunction. I can predict this scene and know how to respond, even though the desperately desired word often hides itself from me also, despite my ardent inferences.

I experience more of this sad and broken reality when Becky and I go out to eat at a particular restaurant. I have not encountered something close to eerie in a restaurant before. It is not the order of the other patrons, who stroll in, order food, talk, pay the bill, go to the restroom, and leave—all without concentration, puzzlement, or difficulty. Yet my wife and I have found an enfeebled order in the disorder. I escort her in, help her get settled, accompany her to the restroom door (sometimes having to convince her she needs help), wait outside, and bring her back to our table, where I order our food and drink and help her use the right utensils. But even this arrangement is subject to disarrangement. Our hard-won islands of coherence are ever threatened by large and looming waves of incoherence. Becky is most fixated on small slivers of purple onion in her salad, favoring them over the lettuce, olives, and other ingredients. This makes no sense, but somehow it fits into a new coherence of incoherence I have learned to accept. In this mental maelstrom, the eerie emerges.

The eerie is different from the merely odd or discomfiting. It is a rude stranger who never becomes a guest. It appears unannounced, unbidden, and cryptically—a ciphered code that is undecipherable. Eeriness is a concept not easily corralled but easily recognized nonetheless. A story featuring an artificially resurrected dead man—part human, part machine—is eerie. Frankenstein's monster does not come selling Girl Scout cookies. His abode is the nightmare or the fictional tale of horror.

Frankenstein is an example of the eerie—and much else. Perhaps a try at definition will articulate the concept. If something (a person, another creature, an event) is eerie, it is at once (1) unexpected, (2) unusual, (3) opaque, and (4) frightening. A letter from a long-lost friend is unexpected, but not eerie. A perfect game in baseball is unusual, but not eerie. The itinerary of subatomic particles is partially opaque, but not eerie. To be alarmed by a barking dog is frightening (at least for a moment), but not eerie. So, it seems we need all four qualifiers to identify the eerie. Frankenstein's monster fulfills all four requirements, as does some of the behavior determined by dementia. Consider more on this.

Unexpected. If eeriness comes on a spectrum, consider the lower levels. My wife now has difficulty putting on her shoes. (At times, so do I. My trouble comes from broken shoelaces, a bad fit, a sore back, or too much girth between me and my feet.) Becky can usually tie her shoelaces; that automatic behavior remains, for a time. She may quickly and firmly tie her laces—but with the shoe on the wrong foot. And I wonder if her successes in matching shoe to foot are now more luck than skill. I never expected this of my wife, so confident in dress and poise and class. Young children can fit a foot to a shoe. Most will do so flawlessly for as long as they have feet and shoes.

Unusual. I knew Becky's abilities would decline, but not the specific order of decay or the timing. Years past, my wife would surprise me (as all spouses do) with an unusual comment or behavior. Becky organized a surprise party to celebrate my getting a doctorate in philosophy. Yet this was nestled in the familiar (and endearing) pattern of our lives. I knew all who yelled "surprise" when I walked in. It was held at a friend's home. Surprise parties are rare and welcomed. The loss of taken-for-granted habits or faculties is never welcomed and often feared. There is nothing to celebrate. It is unusual and unusually distressful.

A retired pastor told me a story about his late father, who had dementia. The pastor looked straight into his father's eyes and said, "Where was your son born?" The father answered perfectly, but had no idea that his son asked the question. This is unusual in a sadly ironic way. The pastor did not use the word *eerie* when recounting the tale, but when I used it to describe the event, his face became serious, thoughtful, and a bit surprised. He did not disagree. We had both beheld the eeriness of dementia.

Opaque. Opacity obscures vision and denies knowledge. In it dwells mysteries and perhaps absurdities. We are normally opaque to one another, at least in some ways. We surprise and even astound each other because of our mutual opacities. As Scripture says, "Each heart knows its own bitterness, / and no one else can share its joy" (Proverbs 14:10). Or as Captain Ahab, an expert on whales, says of the great white whale in *Moby-Dick*, "I shall never know him."

Becky occasionally says things I cannot interpret. It is worse when she is particularly upset, as she often is. These clusters of words are unintelligible and, for now, rare. I can sometimes fill in the gaps and find her intended meaning. Through questions, I discern how the words are switched, the tenses are scrambled, and how the sad Gestalt can be sculpted into intelligibility. As the gap increases between Becky's thoughts and words, so my knowledge of her thoughts decreases.

Some opacity between people can be overcome. The children of Babel are not left with mere babel (Genesis 11). If Chandra speaks only Hindi, I, an American English speaker and a pitiful monolinguist, cannot understand him. But then I call in a translator. Perhaps Chandra or I can learn the other's language. However, no one can translate the languishing language of my wife at her least lucid moments. She knows my language (for now), but all too often I cannot know hers—if there is anything left to know.

Dementia lowers thick, black curtains of opacity, one after another, but at an uneven tempo. Even for a superneurologist—who could fathom the brain's every mystery, and could throw back the curtains of ignorance, and could carefully predict the trajectory of decline—this opacity would remain invincible. No examination, no third-person analysis, can uncover the heart of the self, healthy or unhealthy. No scan can disclose the flickering of this frail light. We are flummoxed by our invincible ignorance. The unfamiliar becomes unavoidable and never settles into a calm pattern.

From one angle, there is no opacity. It is all sickeningly clear. We know that dementia destroys language. But what does she want to say? Why is there no cure? Why did it happen to her and not an evil and bombastic big mouth with millions of fans? There is no unbloodied ignorance in this ongoing tragedy.

I simply cannot know a lot about what Becky thinks and feels. And I am willfully ignorant of some of the specifics of the progression of PPA. It has no cure, and I do not want to further fuel my dread. I know the general outlines, and I know that I will be faced with more events that unravel my sense of normality and unnerve my expectations.

Fear. Last, the eerie elicits a kind of fear or uneasiness. Becky's dementia has not yet caused me to worry about her or my physical safety. That day may come. PPA sufferers can hit and even bite. But apart from that, fear emanates out of unexpected, unusual, and opaque situations. Perhaps fear is too strong a word. The experience is of a disorienting uneasiness, as when someone loses their balance and has to steady themselves quickly to avoid a fall. Becky roams around the house doing things I cannot quite understand; it is unsettling and a bit fearful to me.

Dementia, as I have experienced it, can be eerie. When creation turns against itself at its highest level (human consciousness and speech), the incremental and insidious chaos can rattle the most stable soul.

Five

GIVING UP

DEMENTIA DESTROYS EARTHLY hope since it resists medical cure. At best, dementia might be treated in order to slow down its assault on the brain. When that dread diagnosis is given, all the speculating about symptoms, all the searching for just the right doctor, and all the hopes for a cure vanish in a white hot moment of clarity.

When my wife's psychiatrist said that he and two neurologists identified Becky's disease as primary progressive aphasia, I had never heard of it. (I knew the word *aphasia*, which concerned the loss of speech.) This cruel disorder is a frontal lobe disease. The damage begins in the front of the brain and moves backward, the reverse of Alzheimer's disease. Through a thick Eastern European accent, the dispassionate doctor told me that people live five to ten years after contracting this disease.

At that moment, or not long after, I gave up all hope for my wife's recovery.

For years, I had been managing her decline by trying new doctors, medications, and treatments—and I did not do it that well. We spent thousands of dollars a year on exotic potions and doctors for her manifold ills, which did little if any good. But the wasted money was not the main source of pain. We were crushed by the uncertainty and fatigue of so many failed efforts. I prayed and fasted. We sought out those gifted in healing and spiritual deliverance. We read all the books on healing and labored to implement their admonitions. Yet futility stalked us relentlessly.

But now the verdict was certain, unalterable. The voyage in search of healing ended as the ship of hope sunk into the ocean. Any quixotic quest for any alternative therapy or concoction vanished.

The diagnosis was in. The year before the diagnosis, Becky and I had seen a neurologist who diagnosed depression mimicking dementia. "There is someone in there," he said several times. But he did not know who was in there and misdirected us.

Through that year of futility, the doctor and I interacted a bit about philosophy, since this intrigued him. I wrote a short letter explaining some forms of argument we discussed, using the opportunity to give some logical reasons for Christianity. He was also pleased to receive a copy of my book *Christian Apologetics*. The temptation to retreat into yourself during suffering is great. Looking into the most miserable situations with a desire to find some light makes them more bearable and adds meaning. But after the diagnosis, that was all gone. A threshold had been crossed. Or, I should say, I was dragged across it, since no one takes this trip voluntarily.

Paul Tournier, the Swiss psychiatrist, wrote a book called *To Resist or to Surrender*. Wisdom is proved by knowing when to resist and when to surrender. We should fight against the evils of this world since they flow from the fall of humanity (Genesis 3). However, we often fight battles we find to be futile, and there is no virtue in prolonging the defeat. I had resisted (without denying) Becky's decline for many years. Now I surrendered. Once again, the Preacher of the book of Ecclesiastes gives perspective:

There is a time for everything,
>   and a season for every activity under the heavens:
>   a time to be born and a time to die,
>   a time to plant and a time to uproot,
>   a time to kill and a time to heal,
>   a time to tear down and a time to build,
>   a time to weep and a time to laugh,
>   a time to mourn and a time to dance,
>   a time to scatter stones and a time to gather them,
>   a time to embrace and a time to refrain from embracing,
>   a time to search and a time to give up. (Ecclesiastes 3:1-6)

The concept of a *time* is a recurring theme in Ecclesiastes. God knows the times perfectly, but we mortals do not. Herein lies the *vanity* of our lives. The Preacher is not a nihilist; rather, he is realist. *Vanity* or *meaninglessness* means "vaporous" or "ephemeral."

The Preacher was careful to observe many things, but in all his observations he finds himself hemmed in by ineluctable and exasperating ignorance. The world confounds us too often about too much. And yet, *there is a time to give up*. The wise man, living before God, is more likely to know what time it is than those living otherwise.

Winston Churchill, perhaps the greatest statesman of the twentieth century, famously said, "Never give in—never, never, never, never." When matched against the Nazis in World War II, he was right. Better to go down fighting than to bow to Satan. But dementia is not a Nazi; though it is no less cruel. Unlike the Nazis, dementia cannot be defeated. And to go down fighting an unwinnable war with an indomitable foe is sheer idiocy—and exhausting.

There is a strange release in giving up and giving over, as I did. In her book *Adventures in Prayer*, Catherine Marshall, the Christian devotional writer, drafted a prayer of relinquishment that I often pray and offer to others. Her insights came from a long and painful experience of wrestling with God and his promises.

Father, for such a long time I have pleaded before You this, the deep desire of my heart: [*name your desire here*]. Yet the more I've clamored for Your help with this, the more remote you have seemed.

I confess my demanding spirit in this matter. I've tried suggesting to You ways my prayer could be answered. To my shame, I've even bargained with You. Yet I know that trying to manipulate the Lord of the Universe is utter foolishness. No wonder my spirit is so sore and weary!

I want to trust you, Father. My spirit knows that these verities are forever trustworthy even when I *feel* nothing. . . .

That You are there.

(You said, "Lo, I am with you alway.")

That you love me.

(You said, "I have loved thee with an everlasting love.")

That you alone know what is best for me.

(For in you, Lord, "are hid all the treasures of wisdom and knowledge.")

Perhaps all along, You have been waiting for me to give up self-effort. At last I want You in my life even more than I want [*name your desire here*]. So now, by an act of my will I relinquish this to You. I will accept Your will, whatever that may be. Thank You for counting this act of my will as the decision of the real person even when my emotions protest. I ask You to hold me true to this decision. To You, Lord God, who alone are worthy of worship, I bend the knee with thanksgiving that this too will "work together for good." *Amen*.

The act of giving up frees up possibilities, even though you must accept the unacceptable. There is no utility in futility. When Jesus supernaturally appeared to Saul, who had brutally persecuted Christians, he "heard a voice in Hebrew: 'Saul, Saul, why are you out to get me? Why do you insist on going against the grain?'" (Acts 26:14 *The Message*). The New Living Translation says, "It is useless for you to fight against my will." Going against God's grain is futility without equal. Paul laid down his arms and submitted to Jesus Christ, the good and holy one. Giving in to an illness is different. We surrender to a pox, a plague, a pestilence.

The supreme surrender was that of the Savior to his Father. After his last meal with the disciples (which instituted Communion), Jesus leaned into the *via dolorosa*:

> He withdrew about a stone's throw beyond them, knelt down and prayed, "Father, if you are willing, take this cup from me; yet not my will, but yours be done." An angel from heaven appeared to him and strengthened him. And being in anguish, he prayed more earnestly, and his sweat was like drops of blood falling to the ground. (Luke 22:41-44)

But the greatest life ever lived was not easy to give up, even with the promise of an empty tomb and resurrection ahead. The man who cast out demons with a word, who caused the cripple to dance with joy, who made the blind man see, who gave a widow back her dead son, this man must die—not after a long life, as with Moses, but in his earthly prime. Jesus submitted when he could have escaped.

Yes, I gave up any hope for Becky's healing or for any amelioration of her disease. I would have to manage her decline, day by darkening day. But God had not given up on us, although that often seemed true. In the following pages, I trace this mournful journey of *feeling* so often forsaken, but not *being* forsaken.

> The poor and needy search for water,
>> but there is none;
>> their tongues are parched with thirst.
> But I the Lord will answer them;
>> I, the God of Israel, will not forsake them. (Isaiah 41:17)

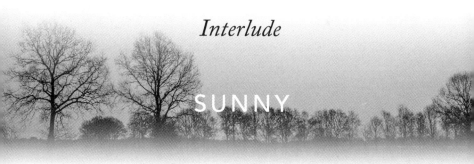

Interlude

SUNNY

ALTHOUGH SHE USUALLY WORKS on Mondays, our live-in care-giver had this Monday off. So, I was responsible for getting Becky's meals. After a morning in the basement reading and giving a radio interview on Descartes and American politics (oddly enough), I realized that Becky needed to be prompted for lunch. So, I went upstairs, with some trepidation. *Trepidation* is my near-constant companion on this journey through twilight.

As I entered her room, I saw a doleful and familiar sight—Becky sitting on the floor weeping. I asked, "What is wrong?" The answer was doleful and familiar as well: "Everything." Sunny had not scurried up the stairs with me, but I knew he would not languish. His ear for crying is well-trained and impeccable. He does not cry, but he knows what our crying is. As he walked in the room, I knew he could comfort Becky without words better than I could comfort her with words.

Sunny is an expert in nuzzling. With his tail wagging low (a sign of nervousness or concern), he put as much of himself on as much of Becky as he was able. One of his best moves is to put his head on the ground while keeping his lower half upright, while making happy sounds and undulating. Sunny rarely does this when he is alone. After nuzzling, licking, and displaying his goldendoodle acrobatics of love, he sat down in front of us, as if to say, "At your service, my humans." Becky and I looked at him, and I sang, "Sunny loves us, this I know, for his licking tells me so." Becky laughed. I laughed. I think Sunny did too.

"Are you ready to have lunch now?" I asked with some confidence. She came down to eat and took two pills meant to calm her. But no pill could substitute for God's grace and comfort-made fur in a dog named Sunny.

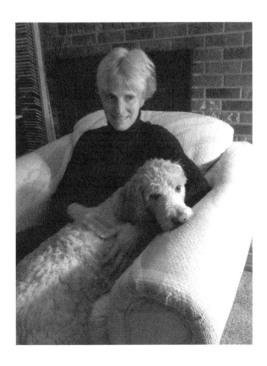

Six

THE TEMPTATION
TO HATE GOD

I AM NOT SURE what event in Becky's decline enraged me more at God. Perhaps it was when I first visited her in a behavioral health unit. Maybe it was an incident that took place shortly after that. Becky had been transferred to another hospital and had been there for only a day or two. I called and asked how she was. "Oh, fine. She is resting after her first ECT."

I screamed into the phone, "What? I did not give permission for that!"

My startled outrage seemed too explosive to be housed in my body. I roared, snorted, lashed out at two innocent objects in the house, and stormed off to the hospital. A bit of sanity slipped into my consciousness, and I stopped by a good friend's house on the way to the hospital. After more yelling, crying, and lamenting the day of my birth (like Job), I settled down a bit and did what I had to do.

ECT means electroconvulsive therapy. It is used to treat extreme depression. Becky and I had been briefed about this a few days earlier by a neurologist who droned on and on with almost no awareness that two shattered souls sat near him. I listened intently, but came to no decision on the treatment, which is nothing like what I saw in the film *One Flew Over the Cuckoo's Nest*, forty years ago. It does not jolt patients into seizures and is very effective. It was right for Becky. But I did not give permission for it.

Livid is too tame a word for how I felt. I called three different doctors as soon as I could about this. They all concurred that ECT was a good idea. I then gave permission for continued treatment. I stopped yelling. I didn't sue anyone. The ECT did help Becky come out of depression. It did nothing to abate her dementia. In fact, it revealed it. If Becky had depression mimicking dementia (which was her earlier diagnosis), the lifting of depression would have restored her cognitive abilities. But it did not.

Part of coming out of my rage was pragmatic, not devotional. I had to decide what to do for the sake of my wife. I had to think clearly. But I did not think dearly of God. Didn't he know I was already overloaded with fear, pain, and sorrow? Didn't he care about my wife, who had been his redeemed child for so long?

I hated God and told him so, repeatedly. I hated myself for doing it, but I did it. But, pragmatically speaking, I needed God's help more than at any other time in my fifty-seven years on earth. I knew rage was of the flesh, not of the Spirit. I never questioned God's existence, only his goodness. I was bordering on misotheism—the "hatred of God." Or maybe I had taken a guest pass into that thought-world. It seemed right, but felt awful. God must have been hearing me, but was not answering—not from a whirlwind or from anywhere else. However, I knew in my bones that God—this mysterious, seemingly heartless God—was my God and that *he was my only hope*. "I will be with [you] in trouble," says he (Psalm 91:15).

I was no model of sanctity while thrashing about in this cauldron of white hot chaos. There was no "peace that passes understanding." What passed understanding was the meaning of these uncharted events. I had let them steal most all of my affection for God. I had lost much of my fear of him as well. I was insolent before the Almighty. My foundations were shaken, but my responsibilities were intensified. The one thing I could not do was ignore God. I am a God-haunted man who knows God and is known by God.

Yet I have a young and brilliant friend who hates God and has no love for him whatsoever. He was raised by godly parents, whose hearts now break for him. I have spoken to and corresponded with this troubled soul. He wrote me one letter (not an email) that was six pages long, typed and single-spaced. He would like to condemn God to hell for the way his family suffered in serving God. I cannot crack his hatred with reason. I wait and pray, and understand some of his rage.

Martin Luther offers me some solace for my tempestuous emotions. A man of courage, intellect, and deep piety, the Reformer was sometimes tempestuous. He reportedly said, "Love God? Sometimes I hate him!" Hating God (episodically) may have its benefits. But, please understand, I do not advise it. Nevertheless, you realize there is a God to be angry with, a God you cannot ignore. And you know God is not ignoring you. Your heart is revealed. No cover-up is possible. When you accuse God, your mood utterly differs from when you love God and sense his love. That sheer juxtaposition of moods may alert you to the fix you are in and drive you back to God in love. I assure you that love is better than hate.

Academics come up with strange and fascinating topics for study. In *Hating God*, Bernard Schweizer named and defined a new religion—or anti-religion—called misotheism. Schweizer defines it as "simply put, misotheism is a response to suffering, injustice, and disorder in a troubled world. Misotheists feel that that humanity is the subject of divine carelessness or sadism, and question God's love for humanity."[1]

Theism, whether Jewish, Christian, or Islamic, confesses a belief in God and accepts (sometimes kicking and screaming) God's authority and prerogatives. Atheism denies the existence of God and tries to live in the aftermath. However, many atheists seem to be proclaiming, "There is no God, and I hate him."

Misotheism denies both theism and atheism. Instead, it accepts the existence of God, but refuses to love, like, or especially *worship* God. Beyond that, misotheists *hate* God, just as misanthropes hate humanity and misogynists hate women. Misotheists shout, "There *is* a God, and I *hate* him." Many of us are *temporary* or *part-time* misotheists. We move from disappointment to irritation to anger and even to outrage at God. I have been guilty of moving past lament and into a noisy (but not dangerous) rage. But these outbursts may escalate beyond short episodes. Sometime after Becky's diagnosis, I handwrote a card to a longtime friend. In it I wrote, "God is cruel, and Ecclesiastes has the courage to admit it." Of course, what prompted this was the ordeal my wife and I were enduring.

As an amateur expert on Ecclesiastes, I thought I was justified in this judgment. Does not the Preacher observe that the unfairness and cruel disappointments of life happen on God's watch?

> Consider what God has done:
>> Who can straighten
>>> what he has made crooked?
>> When times are good, be happy;
>>> but when times are bad, consider this:
>> God has made the one
>>> as well as the other.
>> Therefore, no one can discover
>>> anything about their future. (Ecclesiastes 7:13-14)

"God has made the one as well as the other"—days of joy and days of torment, hours that fly by in joy and hours that crawl along in pain. The Preacher sees God in all events, but he does not turn on God "when times are bad."

After his first round of undeserved suffering, Job agreed with the Preacher, but somehow praised God nonetheless:

> Naked I came from my mother's womb,
>   and naked I will depart.
> The Lord gave and the Lord has taken away;
>   may the name of the Lord be praised. (Job 1:21)

After Job endured his sickness along with the long-winded bad theology of his friends, and after he had made his case against God, God reveals himself and utters a long and irrefutable soliloquy on his supremacy over the animal kingdom. After this drama of divine scolding, Job responds:

> I know that you can do all things;
>   no purpose of yours can be thwarted.
> You asked, "Who is this that obscures my plans
>   without knowledge?"
>   Surely I spoke of things I did not understand,
>   things too wonderful for me to know.
> You said, "Listen now, and I will speak;
>   I will question you,
>   and you shall answer me."
> My ears had heard of you
>   but now my eyes have seen you.
> Therefore I despise myself
>   and repent in dust and ashes. (Job 42:1-6)

Job was humbled. Not all are.

In Dostoevsky's *The Brothers Karamazov*, Ivan Karamazov does not despise himself. He despises God. In the section called "Rebellion," Ivan cites case after case of undeserved human suffering, especially that of children. This is painful to read and to include in this book, but I must, for honesty's sake. Ivan, an irreligious man, confronts his Christian brother, Alyosha. Ivan speaks of

> atrocities being committed all over Bulgaria by the Turks and Circassians, who fear a mass uprising of the Slavs—it appears they set fire to homes and property, they cut people's throats, they rape women and children, they nail prisoners to the palisades by their ears and leave them there until morning, and so on; it really defies imagination. We often talk of man's "bestial" cruelty, but this is terribly unjust and insulting to beasts: a wild animal can never be as cruel as man, as artistic, as refined in his cruelty. The tiger mauls and tears its prey because that is all it knows. It would never enter its head to leave people all night nailed by their ears, even if it could do it. These Turks, incidentally, took a sadistic pleasure in torturing children, starting with cutting them out of their mother's wombs with a dagger, and going so far as to throw babes in arms into the air and impale them on the points of their bayonets before the mother's very eyes.[2]

Ivan, it turns out, is not an atheist. Nor is he a theist. He hates the God who is there and rebels against him. He is a misotheist, and misotheism's most articulate spokesman. He says that no amount of good can compensate for these evils. No greater harmony could justify this kind of man's cruelty to man.

"And that's why I hasten to return my entrance ticket. If I ever want to call myself and honest man, I have to hand it back as soon as possible. And that's exactly what I'm doing. It is not that I don't accept God, Alyosha; I'm just, with utmost respect, handing Him back my ticket."

"That's rebellion," Alyosha said quietly without looking up.[3]

His words haunt me, even as God haunts me more thoroughly. But this Ghost is Holy.

C. S. Lewis was no misotheist, but he was tempted. This is how he expressed shock at God's seeming absence after the death of his wife, Joy Davidman.

When you are happy, so happy you have no sense of needing Him, so happy that you are tempted to feel His claims upon you as an interruption, if you remember yourself and turn to Him with gratitude and praise, you will be—or so it feels—welcomed with open arms. But go to Him when your need is desperate, when all other help is vain, and what do you find? A door slammed in your face, and a sound of bolting and double bolting on the inside. After that, silence.[4]

Lewis was honest with himself and with his readers. He did not lose Christian commitment. He survived his ordeal. But one must read *A Grief Observed* to feel the cost—and benefit—of a thinking man's lament.

When I accuse God of wrongdoing, I do so with a bad conscience, pretending to be righteous. I know too much to really think he is less than perfectly good.[5] But it *feels* as if God were not so. My feelings are not in alignment with divine reality, despite the strength of this rage. I am less than fully sanctified. But when the rage subsides and life ensues, when my wife needs my help and people need to see me strong (even in my weakness), I must return to God.

C. S. Lewis, once again, helped me understand myself in my rage by describing his wrestling with the notion that God might not be good.

> All that stuff about the Cosmic Sadist was not so much the expression of thought as of hatred. I was getting from it the only pleasure a man in anguish can get; the pleasure of hitting back, It was really just . . . mere abuse; "telling God what I thought of Him." And of course, as in all abusive language, "what I thought" didn't mean what I thought true. Only what I thought would offend Him (and His worshippers) most. That sort of thing is never said without some pleasure. Get it "off your chest." You feel better for a moment.[6]

The abuse—God is a sadist!—was for Lewis more an emotional compensation for the agony than it was a settled judgment. I think it was for me as well. Still, the thought comes, *If I were God, I would not allow Becky to suffer so.*

Yet I must also drop the idea that God is an underachiever and that I could do better. How often do we think or say, "If I were God, things would be different!" Some utter this in jest, some out of deep frustration, and some use it as an argument for atheism or misotheism.

First, it is obvious that we are not all-good, all-powerful, and all-knowing. Thus, the idea, "If I were God, I would do X," is absurd, since if you were God you would not be the finite and fallible creature (contingent being) that you are. You cannot just inflate a few of your attributes and claim to occupy the divine throne. You would be revealed as an impostor and kicked off your fake throne.

Second, even though mortals can know many things about God's existence and nature from the Bible, rational intuition, and sound reasoning, much that we would like to know is obscured from us, either by God concealing it or simply because of our finitude. Omniscience has good plans we cannot discern, especially before the plan is achieved. We know in part. God knows in full. We propose means to achieve ends with limited knowledge and virtue. We sometimes succeed and congratulate ourselves or thank God. God knows everything and can bring about whatever he chooses. His means will achieve his ends in his time.

We cry, "If I were God, I would do it better" when our means do not achieve the ends we desire or when we face an intractable evil. Godly people may cry out in lament, "How long, O Lord?" But no person in their right mind would say, "If I were God, I would do it better than God." This is because if you were God, which is impossible, you would do exactly what God has done, is doing, and will do.

I find this argument persuasive, but my emotions may lag behind. I often have to cast myself on Christ's authority and continue to follow him, since there is no other alternative. I want to identify with the apostle Peter, who stuck with Jesus even as others deserted him. The Gospel of John recounts a *hard saying* (as we often put it) of Jesus. In a discourse on salvation, Jesus says,

> Jesus said to them, "Very truly I tell you, unless you eat the flesh of the Son of Man and drink his blood, you have no life in you. Whoever eats my flesh and drinks my blood has eternal life, and I will raise them up at the last day. For my flesh is real food and my blood is real drink. Whoever eats my flesh and drinks my blood remains in me, and I in them. Just as the

living Father sent me and I live because of the Father, so the one who feeds on me will live because of me. This is the bread that came down from heaven. Your ancestors ate manna and died, but whoever feeds on this bread will live forever." He said this while teaching in the synagogue in Capernaum. (John 6:53-59)

When these theological bombshells detonated, they caused casualties. "On hearing it, many of his disciples said, 'This is a hard teaching. Who can accept it?'" (John 6:60).

Jesus did not pander to the crowd, nor did he explain all his teachings at the time he taught.[7] He let these metaphorically pregnant statements stand, and some would not stand for it. After a bit more teaching, we read that

From this time many of his disciples turned back and no longer followed him.

"You do not want to leave too, do you?" Jesus asked the Twelve.

Simon Peter answered him, "Lord, to whom shall we go? You have the words of eternal life. We have come to believe and to know that you are the Holy One of God." (John 6:66-69)

There is no evidence that Peter quite understood this "hard saying." Perhaps he did. But despite the departure of "many of his disciples," Peter remained. He had to stay because he knew Jesus, who had shown himself to be true and reliable. Peter accompanied Jesus and beheld his teachings, his miracles, and his loving and just character. Where else could Peter go? This, of course, was Peter at his best. He is known for some wide faith fluctuations, at least before Pentecost. But his testimony tells us this: we can live wisely within ignorance if it is bracketed by knowledge.[8] Hundreds of years before, the Preacher told us (and I come back to his words so often),

> When I applied my mind to know wisdom and to observe the labor that is done on earth—people getting no sleep day or night—then I saw all that God has done. No one can comprehend what goes on under the sun. Despite all their efforts to search it out, no one can discover its meaning. Even if the wise claim they know, they cannot really comprehend it. (Ecclesiastes 8:16-17)

If we are tempted to look elsewhere for meaning and hope in this suffering, we must return to the earnest confession of Peter: "Where else can we go?" Like Peter, I know too much to go back. I cannot become an atheist, a Buddhist, a Hindu, a new ager, a Muslim, a misotheist, or even an agnostic. I know too much to go back. As the simple gospel song says, "I have decided to follow Jesus. No turning back. No turning back."

I cannot leave Jesus permanently. My trust waxes and wanes, but unlike the routine of the tides, it is unpredictable. Unlike Peter, I have not denied Jesus before others, but like a fool I have told God off in the presence of another. When I am outraged at God, I try to think of God in Christ hanging on a cross for me. This sometimes brings me back to theological and psychological sanity if not sanctity. I must work with what I have and seek more as I walk through an ever-darkening twilight.

The best way to hate God is on your knees (literally or in your heart), hoping that hate will be transformed into submissive love in the divine presence. Surely, this Godward accusation is better than indifference or apathy. As William Backus argued, most Christians have a "hidden rift with God," which God wants to take away.[9] But some of us have an open and bleeding and wide rift with God. Like the patriarch Jacob, we should wrestle with God until he blesses us. The blessing, however, always comes with a wound (Genesis 33:22-32), and we limp along until we rise again, never to limp again.

Seven

LEARNING TO LAMENT

As BLAISE PASCAL noted in his *Pensées,*

> All men seek happiness. There are no exceptions. However different the means they may employ, they all strive towards this goal. The reason why some go to war and some do not is the same desire in both, but interpreted in two different ways. This will never takes the least step except to that end. This is the motive of every act of every man, including those who go and hang themselves.[1]

Our question, our cry of the wounded heart, is whether some mode of happiness can be kept in the face of keen suffering.[2] Pascal offered no snake oil. He knew how to lament while retaining his Christian convictions, as evidenced in his essay "Prayer to Ask of God the Proper Use of Suffering."[3] Suffering, wisely born through lament, can yield meaning, but this wins little applause in American culture.

A vast literature on happiness has emerged in recent years based on "positive psychology." Instead of emphasizing neurosis and disorders, psychologists are exploring what leads to human fulfillment. One book I have read is called *Authentic Happiness* and is based on careful research on what makes people happy.[4] That is good in its place, but we have little instruction on the wise use of woe. There is, to my knowledge, no book called *Authentic Sadness*. However, I read one called *Against Happiness*.

Throughout this doleful and, I hope, hopeful book, I have lamented much over all the losses that have assailed Becky and me. Nevertheless, my reflections have an aim: to live well with suffering in light of reality in God's world. I want to extend those reflections here in more detail. G. K. Chesterton said that he spent his entire career opposing two heresies, optimism and pessimism. The third way is hope. Paul knew that hope is refined through tribulation, and that tribulation can be endured through hope.

> We . . . glory in our sufferings, because we know that suffering produces perseverance; perseverance, character; and character, hope. And hope does not put us to shame, because God's love has been poured out into our hearts through the Holy Spirit, who has been given to us. (Romans 5:3-5)

Hope is a discipline that can be cultivated and even celebrated. I take it that hope—grounded in truth—needs lament as its tonic. Hope, if hard won, both consoles and inspires. But nobody needs hope on the cheap. There are carnival barkers and snake oil peddlers galore who offer nothing but prevarication that trades on desperation. Hope proffered at the expense of fact is cruel. It only adds deception to sorrow. We should avoid taking harbor in what ends up being a sewer.

Christians acknowledge the tragic dimensions of life. Unlike new agers, Christian Scientists, ethical relativists, and postmodernists, we believe that evil things happen. They are not illusions of our befogged minds; real evil cannot be redescribed to soften its bite. Ever since the fall of humanity, the world has been beset with death,

decay, and disappointment (Genesis 3; Romans 3), so much so that
Paul says the entire universe groans in travail until its final liberation:
"We know that the whole creation has been groaning as in the pains
of childbirth right up to the present time. Not only so, but we
ourselves, who have the firstfruits of the Spirit, groan inwardly as we
wait eagerly for our adoption to sonship, the redemption of our
bodies" (Romans 8:22-23).

We cannot be Pollyannas and manufacture cheap consolation and
pseudocomfort in order to shield ourselves or others from the
emotional depths of loss. There are inscrutable evils in this fallen
world that cannot be papered over by trite or sentimental comments.

Virtuously aligning human feeling with objective fact is no small
endeavor, and it takes us far beyond pleasurable sensations. As
C. S. Lewis wrote in *The Abolition of Man*,

> Until quite modern times all teachers and even all men be-
> lieved that universe to be such that certain emotional reac-
> tions on our part could either be congruous or incongruous
> to it—believed, in fact, that object did not merely receive,
> but could merit, our approval or disapproval, our reverence
> or out contempt.[5]

If Lewis is right, then some objects and situations in this fallen
world merit lament as well. But our affections are too often out of
gear. We often weep when we should laugh and laugh when we
should weep. Or we feel nothing when we should feel something.
Decades ago, a pop song confessed, "Sometimes I don't know what
to feel."[6] We have all felt this confusion. I often feel this with my
wife, since so many of her moods, thoughts, and behaviors are bizarre,
and I have little experience in ministering to her like this. We live

in-between times and "under the sun," as Ecclesiastes puts it. Accordingly, we are obligated to know what time it is.

> There is a time for everything,
>> and a season for every activity under the heavens: . . .
>> a time to weep and a time to laugh,
>> a time to mourn and a time to dance. (Ecclesiastes 3:1, 4)

Sadness has its seasons, as does happiness; this is simply because God's creation has fallen into sin and has yet to reach its culmination in the new heaven and the new earth (Revelation 21–22). Before then, we are still exiles (1 Peter 2:11). If we are to be wise stewards of our emotions, we must know the signs of the times, know our present time, and know what these times should elicit within us.

Our sadness should be judicious and obedient, not hasty, melodramatic, or inane. This is a moral and spiritual matter, not one of mere feelings. Emotions easily err. After the Colorado Rockies baseball team was eliminated from a playoff game some years ago, a Rockies fan reported that this loss was like "a death in the family." That struck me as pathetic, if not daft—the sadness of a disordered soul. I wonder how her family members responded to this. One can care too little or too much about anything. Sentimentality may be defined as caring for something more than God does. This is the open secret of idolatry.

Sadness intrudes unbidden in a variety of dark shades. I cannot offer a taxonomy or hierarchy of it here. Rather, consider one often-misunderstood form of sorrow—lament. What is it? Frederick Buechner wrote in *Wishful Thinking: A Seeker's ABC*: "The place God calls you to is the place where your deep gladness and the world's deep hunger meet." In that spirit, lament is where our deep sadness meets the world's deep wounds. And this world has its wounds. Even God Incarnate bears wounds, his and ours.

Many impugn God's allowance of evil by claiming that God is far removed from our earthly turmoil. But he is not. No other God bears scars—the scars of crucifixion, of rejection, of betrayal, and of humiliation. Jesus Christ knows our pain from the inside out because he suffered more than any human being in the history of the universe. He is our high priest only because he sank so low as to submit to death on a cruel Roman cross for crimes he did not commit (Philippians 2:5-11). God not only *sympathizes* with us, he *empathizes* with us.

The deepest wound of all wounds was the crucifixion of the Lord Jesus Christ, who suffered more than anyone ever had or ever will, and with the greatest possible effect. His cry was the apex of all laments: "My God, my God, why have you forsaken me?" (Matthew 27:46; see Psalm 22:1). It is only because of this lament that our laments gain their ultimate meaning. If the perfect Son of God can lament and not sin, so may we. Further, that anguished cry was answered by his resurrection from the dead on the third day.

But Christ looked ahead to his and our resurrection and gave us a model.

> And let us run with perseverance the race marked out for us, fixing our eyes on Jesus, the pioneer and perfecter of faith. For the joy set before him he endured the cross, scorning its shame, and sat down at the right hand of the throne of God. Consider him who endured such opposition from sinners, so that you will not grow weary and lose heart. (Hebrews 12:1-3)

Christians lament because objective goods have been violated or destroyed. Creation is deemed good by God himself (Genesis 1). Yet humans have rebelled against God, themselves, each other, and creation. As the Preacher puts it, "All things are wearisome, / more than one can say" (Ecclesiastes 1:8). In *Lament for a Son*, Nicholas Wolterstorff notes that Jesus blesses those who mourn (Matthew 5:4) because they are "aching visionaries" seeking genuine goods that escape their grasp. In this sense, their godly frustration is their blessing—and the aching will one day be answered. Wolterstorff's profound words demand to be quoted in full.

> Who then are the mourners? The mourners are those who have caught a glimpse of God's new day, who ache with all their being for that day's coming, and who break out into tears when confronted with its absence. They are the ones who realize that in God's realm of peace there is no one blind and who ache whenever they see someone unseeing. They are the ones who realize that in God's realm there is no one hungry and who ache whenever they see someone starving. They are the ones who realize that in God's realm there is no one falsely accused and who ache whenever they see someone imprisoned unjustly. They are the ones who realize that in God's realm there is no one who fails to see God and who ache whenever they see someone unbelieving. They are the ones who realize that in God's realm there is no one who suffers oppression and who ache whenever they see someone beat down. They are the ones who realize that in God's realm there is no one without dignity and who ache whenever they see someone treated with indignity. They are the ones who realize that in God's realm of peace there is neither death nor tears and who ache whenever they see someone crying tears over death. The mourners are aching visionaries.[7]

When we lament, we do not do so in a void of meaninglessness. Even though many of our desires are disordered, and thus vain or evil, a good many of them remain in line with God's desire to restore shalom. We cry out over the loss of a child, over war, over stupidity, cupidity, mortality, dementia, and more. Paul was in anguish over the unbelief of his countrymen: "I have great sorrow and unceasing anguish in my heart. For I could wish that I myself were cursed and cut off from Christ for the sake of my people, those of my own race, the people of Israel" (Romans 9:2-4; see also Romans 10:1). But Paul never descended into despair or gave up the cause of Christ. Even having suffered terrible torments for Christ, he marched on, knowing that the End puts all the means into place and that our "labor in the Lord is not in vain" (1 Corinthians 15:58).

Lament is not only a literary genre of Scripture (consider the many psalms of lament, such as 22, 39, 88, and 90, as well the book of Lamentations); it is an indelible category of human existence east of Eden and under the sun.[8] It can be done well or poorly, but it cannot be avoided by any but sociopaths. Fallen mortals bemoan life's suffering, often mixing their grief with outrage. Whether outwardly or only inwardly, they raise their voices, shake their fists, beat their breasts, and shed hot tears.

The Negro spiritual intones, "Nobody knows the trouble I've seen. Nobody knows but Jesus." Or listen to the contralto Marian Anderson sing, "Were You There When They Crucified My Lord?" The blues, leaning on the spirituals, lament in a thousand ways. "Nobody knows you when you're down and out," cries Eric Clapton.[9] When Duke Ellington played his wordless lament "Mood Indigo" on his first European tour, some in the audience wept. Even heavy metal, full of thunder, rage, and debauchery, often laments life's burdens with pain-soaked shouts.

In Metallica's "Master of Puppets," leader singer James Hetfield's voice is that of cocaine. It lies, enslaves, manipulates, and pulls the strings of the addicted. This is a roaring, electronic lament. But there is no hope. It is protest without promise. Still, I often listen to it and other pieces by this loud, angry, and sometimes profound group. Metallica, at its best, draws one into a fellowship of the fall, if not redemption. But that can make redemption all the more sweet.[10]

If I have established something of the meaning of lament biblically and philosophically, I need delve into its practice in this world of woe and wonder, of weeping and laughing, of mourning and dancing (Ecclesiastes 3:1-8).

First, those who take the Bible to be the knowable revelation of God about the things that matter most should discover the genre of lament in Scripture. Besides the psalms of lament and Lamentations, perhaps Ecclesiastes is the richest biblical resource. The Preacher is weighed down by the seeming futility of life but realizes that sadness gives needed, if unwanted, lessons.

> It is better to go to a house of mourning
>   than to go to a house of feasting,
> for death is the destiny of everyone;
>   the living should take this to heart.
> Frustration is better than laughter,
>   because a sad face is good for the heart.
> The heart of the wise is in the house of mourning,
>   but the heart of fools is in the house of pleasure.
>   (Ecclesiastes 7:2-4)

Joy has its lessons, but mourning has lessons that only mourning can teach. Better to be its attentive students than delinquents who avoid the duties and gifts of "the sad face." Francis Schaeffer, one of the key figures of twentieth-century Christianity, was known for his *sad eyes*. But sadness did not override compassion or passion for truth, God, Scripture, or people. He rejoiced greatly when someone converted, and celebrated by playing the Hallelujah Chorus on his phonograph at high volume.

Ecclesiastes, more than any other book of Holy Scripture, has given me the perspective and language of lament necessary for my own sad sojourn during the last fifteen or so years with my chronically and now mentally ill wife. It is a deep well of tough wisdom for the weary and wasted soul.

Second, lament requires a deep knowledge of God, of the world, and of ourselves. It is often said that our hearts should break where God's heart breaks. We should "rejoice with those who rejoice; mourn with those who mourn" (Romans 12:15). Mourning rightly is a rare skill and one that cannot be cultivated without the sacrifice of one's ego on behalf of another soul and God. Any hospital chaplain worth having must develop this art of sympathy and empathy. But we are all chaplains in the hospice of life.

To adjust our emotions to reality, we must gain knowledge from the Bible and sound thinking (Romans 12:1-2). We are not to grieve the Holy Spirit (Ephesians 4:30). A corollary is that we should know what grieves the Holy Spirit, and grieve along with him.

Third, our grieving and our hoping find their meaning in our knowledge of God. But we can also rest in our ignorance of some of his ways. We do well to remember the limits of our understanding as finite and fallen creatures. Job was never given a specific answer as to why God allowed the devil to torment him. Instead, God revealed his own greatness and power, and asked Job to trust him in that light (Job 38–42). This does not mean the Bible advises intellectual capitulation, because God does invite us to "reason together" with him (Isaiah 1:18 KJV) and to give a reason for the hope that we have (1 Peter 3:15). It is reasonable to suppose that the ways of an all-powerful and all-knowing God will sometimes be mysterious to us.

But these unsearchable paths of God—the thick, dark, heavy mysteries of providence—are not absurdities; they are not meaningless. Their meaning is, however, largely opaque to us now. But God promised his children that "in all things God works for the good of those who love him, who have been called according to his purpose" (Romans 8:28). There is meaning in these events, even if much of that meaning now escapes us.

Fourth, biblical lament is not grumbling, which is selfish, impatient, and pointless. The children of Israel grumbled against God even as God was providing for their pilgrimage, just as he promised. Paul says, "Do everything without grumbling or arguing" (Philippians 2:14). While the distinction between grumbling and lament is not easy to make, it is a real distinction, since Scripture encourages lament and warns against grumbling. Isaiah declares a lament was needed:

The Lord, the LORD Almighty,
     called you on that day
to weep and to wail,
     to tear out your hair and put on sackcloth. (Isaiah 22:12)

Last, we lament when God seems silent and distant. We lament before the face of God, however distant he seems. C. S. Lewis puts this principle into the voice of a senior demon in *The Screwtape Letters*. Perhaps no one has said it better: "Be not deceived, Wormwood, our cause is never more in danger than when a human, no longer desiring, but still intending, to do our Enemy's will, looks round upon a universe in which every trace of Him seems to have vanished, and asks why he has been forsaken, and still obeys."[11]

I have found that no matter how distant God may seem, no matter how unendurable my situation has become, no matter how angry with God I am, it will not always be so. God brings good times and bad times. If we know Jesus as our Lord and the Lord of history and eternity, then we can endure because the love God gives us "always protects, always trusts, always hopes, always perseveres" (1 Corinthians 13:7). One day, we shall prevail. "If God is for us, who can be against us?" (Romans 8:31). But how deeply and how often do we feel this, experience it emotionally?

Some Christian writers—and wise ones—counsel us to learn to enjoy God, to experience the joy of his promises and the certainty we have of his love written in blood by Jesus.[12] I agree. And yet I seldom find emotional help here. The truth I know. The Bible I read. My Savior is real. The Spirit leads. And yet I more often endure than I exult. And yet—what is to come is better than what is now. God will lift up those who mourn and grieve before him. "Blessed are those who mourn, / for they will be comforted" (Matthew 5:4).

The Bible endorses lament, but it is better known for endorsing and encouraging joy, even "joy unspeakable and full of glory" (1 Peter 1:8 KJV). Sadly, I am no expert on joy, although I find meaning and some happiness in many things. However, I can endeavor to "set [my] heart on things above" (Colossians 3:1) and to remember God's power and goodness. Memorizing Scripture is no small comfort in this (Psalm 119:11). I often repeat to myself:

> Truly my soul finds rest in God;
>> my salvation comes from him.
> Truly he is my rock and my salvation;
>> he is my fortress, I will never be shaken. (Psalm 62:1-2)

We must turn and return to the Holy Scriptures to rightly orient ourselves every day to every condition of life. And that Bible comforts only with truth, but what comfort it is.

The triune God will judge and resurrect the entire cosmos in the end (Daniel 12:2; Matthew 25:31-46; John 5; Revelation 20–22). On this, we place our trust and direct our hope. Future grace awaits us. Yet the Lamb then in our midst was once scarred and suffered for us by his Father's will for the sake of our redemption. God counts our tears before he takes them away (Psalm 56:8; Revelation 21:4). Learning to lament is, then, part of our lot under the sun. We and our neighbors are better for it, tears and all.

Interlude

MY WORRIED EAR

FOR YEARS I HAVE HAD A WORRIED EAR. I do not mean tinnitus or hearing loss. It is worse than that. My hearing is fine, but what I often hear is not. I hear the sounds of distress, confusion, or anger. These are the sounds of dementia.

As my wife grew worse physically and emotionally, I became worried about what I heard in our home. Our home since 2013 has very thin floors. Sounds spread easily from floor to floor. Was that a cry? Is she wandering around needing help, or is it our caregiver tiding up before she goes to bed? I turn down the music and listen hard, orienting my whole body toward perceiving and interpreting sounds. Is that Becky coming down the stairs (again) and lightly stepping around the corner? Sometimes, I am prepared; other times, I am not. Sunny may come over to my chair before Becky and nuzzle me nervously. He knows that Becky is coming and wants to warn me.

I get spooked when she appears silently, troubled, and unable to say why. It is eerie, eerie. As I type, I hear ambiguous noises again. Will she appear before me mute and pathetic, looking to me for what I cannot give her—assurance, hope, and peace? Although I richly enjoy listening to music through my headphones, I seldom put them on. Too many times has the music been interrupted when I am startled by poor Becky.

This is my worried ear.

Eight

JOY IN LAMENT

SUFFERING COMES IN MANY FACES, and no one can penetrate into the inner sanctum of another's woes (Proverbs 14:12). However, we all share in suffering and often suffer together. We can learn how to suffer well from others who suffer from different ills than we do (see Hebrews 11). We can also avoid the errors in suffering that we see others commit (see 1 Corinthians 10:1-22). We all need models of virtue to emulate and examples of vice to eschew. Paul says this of the Old Testament writings: "Everything that was written in the past was written to teach us, so that through the endurance taught in the Scriptures and the encouragement they provide we might have hope" (Romans 15:4).

One of the happiest men I know moves about in a high tech and outrageously expensive wheelchair (to use an outmoded term). He has not walked on his own for over thirty years and needs help getting up, bathing, and going to bed. Stuart needs several male assistants working for him. He befriends all of his helpers and becomes their spiritual mentor. This is Stuart Smith, one of my best and oldest friends.

I met Stuart in 1979, just after I graduated from the University of Oregon in Eugene. Stuart pastored a small congregation, Orchard Community Church. I met with Stuart shortly after beginning to attend and helped him walk during his work breaks. I would lift him out of his chair and then give my arm to steady him as he bravely swung his legs into a halting but confident gate. My sadness over Stuart's plight (a rare muscle-degenerating disease) was more than matched by his humble, gentle, and loving spirit.

Stuart was my pastor for five years. He was an able teacher, both in the pulpit and in the rest of his life. He also worked as an editor for many years and edited my doctoral dissertation (for free). Oddly, Becky's editing prowess and my adviser's sensibilities did not synchronize.

I have only seen Stuart angry once. A number of couples in our church had divorced in the early 1980s, forcing Stuart to preach on this. Without rancor or bitterness, he read loudly and firmly from Malachi 2:16, which condemns divorce. Jesus, of course, was angry at sin as well (Matthew 23).

My friend has suffered physical problems unknown to most mortals. He has little physical strength left. But his mind is sharp and his heart is warm. He has asked God for healing from the disease, and God has not given it. God has answered many other prayers, some of them prayers related to Stuart's health. Most people with his condition die long before Stuart's age. Many with debilitating illnesses die spiritually, becoming bitter and angry at everything.

Stuart has suffered through more than physical debility, some of it crushing. (After a family crisis, he cried for hours and hours for weeks on end.) But Stuart does not get by through mere optimism. When I have confided in him about my suffering, he has never given me easy answers. Instead, he commiserates, counsels, and cares. He prays for me. I pray for him.

Stuart continues to study and write. I recently endorsed his book *Dead to Sin, Alive to God*, an insightful study on the Christian life.[1] To write such a book—or any book—when he cannot type, turn the pages of a book, or pull a book off the shelf is remarkable, inspiring, and praiseworthy.

One might say that Stuart was gifted with a more cheerful disposition than I have. He is not melancholic. I sometimes ooze melancholy. But Stuart would credit all his joy and strength to God. He lives a deep spiritual life and often derives deep insights from Scripture. He knows what the dark and deep pit looks like, from the inside. But he has never remained there. Stuart can affirm with the psalmist:

> He lifted me out of the slimy pit,
>   out of the mud and mire;
> he set my feet on a rock
>   and gave me a firm place to stand. (Psalm 40:2)

But because his Lord Jesus Christ enables Stuart Smith to *stand firm* even in his enfeebled body, I am inspired to *stand firm* (as I wait) through my laments.

Now, Not Yet
by Douglas Groothuis

Blank walls
    When signs are needed.
Dark ceilings
    When skylights are dreamt of.
Hard walls
    When there must be windows.
A rose crushed

Against the bottom of a garbage can.
Walking
    In circles, circles . . .
    Circles.
Running
    Uphill, breathless (hopelessly hoping yet)
Waiting
    In the hospice of life
        For the joy that promises deathless to come.

Nine

MOSES AND OUR SADNESS

MOSES WROTE BUT ONE PSALM. He had the credentials as the lawgiver, a prophet, a man who led God's people out of Egypt, a man who saw God and lived, and a man who was barred from entering the Promised Land because of his irresponsible anger. Moses was a man of deep feeling and insight. He knew how to lament before the God of Israel. Another psalm tells us that "He [God] made known his ways to Moses, / his deeds to the people of Israel" (Psalm 103:7).

This man of God wrote a psalm to teach us how to lament before the God we wrestle with so often. I have preached this psalm many times, and each time I am jolted by its honesty, hope, wisdom, and even audacity. I offer a few words on Psalm 90 in light of my walk through twilight with Becky.

The psalms are prayers that express the full gamut of human emotions. They are God's prayer book for humanity and for every situation in life. This psalm is Moses' poetic reflection on his epic life.

Lord, you have been our dwelling place
    throughout all generations.
Before the mountains were born
    or you brought forth the whole world,
    from everlasting to everlasting you are God. (Psalm 90:1-2)

Whatever else happens and whatever we feel, we can know that we dwell in God's world, even in God's home. All generations have shared this divine envelopment. God was there eternally before he created the cosmos and will be there "from everlasting to everlasting." The mountains, a symbol of the ancient, are not older than their Creator. Moses' ringing affirmations are the foundation for what follows: we are God's creatures and we live with him, come what may.

I can get so snagged by a hundred caregiver anxieties and my guilt over things left undone and things done wrongly that I forget the truths of verses 1-2. God is before all, he transcends us as Creator, he brought forth nature and humanity to dwell in him—but as dust. Although we dwell in God, a chasm emerges between the creature and the Creator.

> You turn people back to dust,
>   saying, "Return to dust, you mortals."
> A thousand years in your sight
>   are like a day that has just gone by,
>   or like a watch in the night. (Psalm 90:3-4)

The residents of God's house are dust people who return to dust at the command of the deity. By command we exist; by command we return to dust. At some point all of us lose our youth and sense the dustiness of ourselves. When Becky and I married, I knew our health and gifts were not everlasting on this earth. We were not in decline, but in our prime. We didn't smell or taste or feel any dust, and it did not get in our starry eyes. But, as the Preacher says, "time and chance happens to them all" (Ecclesiastes 9:11).

In our time, we are ephemeral dust before an eternal God. For God, a millennium is like "a yesterday" and a mere "watch in the night," which was three or four hours. God is "the Ancient of Days"

(Daniel 7:22). Our days are numbered, and numbered by God. Pascal seeks to arouse a soul-sleeping world by this parable:

> Imagine a number of men in chains, all under sentence of death, some of whom are each day butchered in the sight of the others; those remaining see their own condition in that of their fellows, and looking at each other with grief and despair await their turn. This is an image of the human condition.[1]

In *Being Mortal*, surgeon Atul Gawande observes that doctors are trained to fix the body. They are neither trained nor skilled in managing the mortality of their patients, since a dying patient is a failure for the doctor.[2] But he argues that there is more to life than length of days.

For one afflicted with severe dementia or any horrible illness, the gray and black days move at a glacial pace. Each day is closer to eternity, closer to joining the Ancient of Days, in whose presence time has no curse. But we cannot blame those suffering in this way if they yearn for death. Suicide is never an option, but wanting to die when the days are curses and when our mind and senses betray us is understandable. Moses himself wanted to die, so heavy was the weight of leading God's people: "I cannot carry all these people by myself; the burden is too heavy for me. If this is how you are going to treat me, please go ahead and kill me—if I have found favor in your eyes—and do not let me face my own ruin" (Numbers 11:14-15). God answered his anguished prayer by giving him the strength to lead God's people. But the man who felt this way knows how to lament, and Moses is not done lamenting in this psalm. More metaphors remind us of the dust we are:

> Yet you sweep people away in the sleep of death—
>   they are like the new grass of the morning:

> In the morning it springs up new,
>> but by evening it is dry and withered. (Psalm 90:5-6)

The residents of God's own home have no security in their mortality. They are washed away and die. They spring up with green promise and wither away as gray death and dust. Dementia withers the mind, and is all the more tragic for a mind like Becky's that sprouted up as brilliant in youth, became more brilliant as it matured, expressed that brilliance through writing, editing, and speaking, and then withers, not quickly, but slowly. Moses would have understood. But it gets worse for poor mortals.

> We are consumed by your anger
>> and terrified by your indignation.
> You have set our iniquities before you,
>> our secret sins in the light of your presence.
>> (Psalm 90:7-8)

Morality now confronts mortality. God is angry with his houseguests because they have committed iniquities before him. To those attending to God and their consciences, this should dismay us deeply and consume our consciousness. The sins we hide from others are transparent to the transcendent. Iniquities that are locked down or covered up are brought up and held up by the everlasting One. A politician may have his key documents legally sealed, but Jesus breaks open all seals in his time. These seals are but dust—dust hiding dust.

Moses exposes the gap between God and humanity by naming God as Creator and everlasting as compared to being a creature who is ephemeral. He introduces into the psalm a moral breach. Since he wrote the book of Genesis, Moses knows that man and woman were expelled out of the garden because of their rebellion against

God in succumbing to the serpent's seductions (Genesis 3:1-6).
Given his life of confronting the evils of Pharaoh and the waywardness
of the children of Israel, Moses would agree with David's plea for
forgiveness after his egregious sins of adultery and murder.

> I know my transgressions,
>> and my sin is always before me.
> Against you, you only, have I sinned
>> and done what is evil in your sight;
> so you are right in your verdict
>> and justified when you judge.
> Surely I was sinful at birth,
>> sinful from the time my mother conceived me.
>> (Psalm 51:3-5)

As I have walked, and often stumbled, through this involuntary
path of lament, I have acted dishonorably in my rage and terror. I
would rather not tell everyone the full story of my response to
Becky's tragedy. Yet God knows, and knows I am dust.

> He knows how we are formed,
>> he remembers that we are dust. (Psalm 103:14)

Moses continues to lament. He will not muffle the voice of
our suffering.

> All our days pass away under your wrath;
>> we finish our years with a moan.
> Our days may come to seventy years,
>> or eighty, if our strength endures;
> yet the best of them are but trouble and sorrow,
>> for they quickly pass, and we fly away.
> If only we knew the power of your anger!

> Your wrath is as great as the fear that is your due.
>> (Psalm 90:9-11)

The New Revised Standard Version makes verse 9 more clear when it says,

> For all our days pass away under your wrath;
>> our years come to an end like a sigh.

Moses knew of God's gracious covenants and the gifts he bestowed on his people. Moses knew that wrath is not all there is to God. Yet wrath remains.

> God is a righteous judge,
>> a God who displays his wrath every day. (Psalm 7:11)

Moses beheld the judgments of God on Egypt and on the children of Israel, yet he did not fathom the severity of judgment; neither did Abraham, King David, or any mere mortal.

Even a good, long life of seventy to eighty years—Moses lived to be one hundred and twenty—cannot compensate for the ills of fleeting pride, labor, and sorrow. Moses, man of God, is morose.

The average age of death differs from time to time and place to place, but I am about a decade from seventy. Becky is older. Unlike Christopher Hitchens (d. 2012), reporter extraordinaire, atheist provocateur, prolific author, and acerbic commentator and debater, I do not write as one without hope of the afterlife, as he did in *Mortality*.[3] We are hopeful grasshoppers. We drag ourselves along, but toward a finish line, which is the portal to eternal felicity (Ecclesiastes 12:1-5).

But what of God's wrath and anger? Is this not dispiriting and dreadful? Moses addressed God and beseeched God in this prayer. He did not recoil into silence or screaming. How much more for Becky and me, iniquitous mortals who nevertheless know the name of our Savior? Only Christ experienced the full effect of God's anger against sin when he became a sin offering for sinners. "God made him who had no sin to be sin for us, so that in him we might become the righteousness of God" (2 Corinthians 5:21).

Becky and I are made in the divine image: we are sinners and we are redeemed through the work of Jesus Christ. If we cannot divine the meaning of why providence has dealt us dementia, we can understand the forgiveness we need and have been given. Moses now implores God in light of the agony he has described.

> Teach us to number our days,
>> that we may gain a heart of wisdom. (Psalm 90:12)

Because of our sad lot in God's house, our days are numbered. But not all number their days. Many live carelessly, thinking of themselves as immortal. A terminal disease or dementia changes that quickly. Primary progressive aphasia is a terminal disease, and its countdown is vague and vexing. The time bomb is ticking, but I cannot clearly hear the ticks. Eventually, if she does not expire from another malady, Becky's brain will cease to tell her body how to live at all. She is dying, but slowly. Becky made good use of her time before all this. She made a good mark on this unholy world.

I have pondered verse 12 for decades. Now it shines brighter and penetrates deeper into me, the aging grasshopper. I beg God that my days outnumber my wife's days, since I need to take care of her. But my calling is not muted by this suffering. The following verse challenged me to finish my large book *Christian Apologetics*, and it continues to urge me on, no matter what. Paul instructs, "Tell Archippus: 'See to it that you complete the ministry you have received in the Lord'" (Colossians 4:17).

Christian faith, when well-practiced, is incompatible with the panic of fearfully rushing on lest time run out. Yet there is urgency to my work as a teacher, preacher, and writer. Becky and I felt this for years as we spent vacation time researching and writing books. I took as many speaking engagements as I could. We are meaning-driven people. The days of articles, books, and public speaking are over for my once-brilliant wife. They are not over for her husband, and I soldier on. I take heart in Paul's words: "Continue to work out your salvation with fear and trembling, for it is God who works in you to will and to act in order to fulfill his good purpose" (Philippians 2:12-13).

Now Moses opens wider his broken heart to the Almighty, imploring him to bless in four more ways.

> Relent, LORD! How long will it be?
>> Have compassion on your servants. (Psalm 90:13)

Moses passionately requests that God return in blessing, in light of the curses he describes. The word translated "return" is close to *repent*. Moses is exhorting the God in whom he and we dwell to *finally* show sorrow for his servants in tangible ways. The psalms often cry to God "How long?" (Psalm 6:3; 13:1). How I feel this in my soul. I am exhausted from waiting for relief. For years, I sought God through prayer, fasting, and claiming portions of Scripture to bring healing for Becky. But, as I said earlier, I have given up on that. But I still cry, "How long will it be" until God returns in blessing and his compassion is more evident? I unite with Moses in more entreaties.

> Satisfy us in the morning with your unfailing love,
>> that we may sing for joy and be glad all our days.
> Make us glad for as many days as you have afflicted us,
>> for as many years as we have seen trouble.
>> (Psalm 90:14-15)

In about 2008 I began to pray these verses earnestly. This was before Becky's dementia. But I told God that we had been afflicted enough by Becky's illnesses and other sorrows. It was a heavy weight and not getting lighter. We needed joy. I thus asked God for ten or fifteen years of gladness "according to the days" he had afflicted us and "the years we had seen evil." It seemed a fair request. It certainly was an earnest one. I memorized most of Psalm 90 and prayed it repeatedly. Life went on in meaningful ways. I was writing, teaching, and preaching. But the pressures of Becky's ill health did not subside; they got worse. When Becky was given the verdict of dementia, that prayer ended. No earthly compensation would be made for the affliction and evil sent to us.

God has doubtless sometimes answered this prayer by making the later seasons of life better than the early ones. A good friend tells me that he is enjoying and thriving in his ministry of speaking and writing more in his seventies than at any other time. And we are told that "the LORD blessed the latter part of Job's life more than the former part" (Job 42:12). Perhaps it will be so for me, somehow; but apart from a miracle, it will not be so for Becky. We must transfer our hopes to the new world that is coming. The days of glory will endlessly dwarf those of misery. "Amazing Grace" sums it up.

> When we've been there ten thousand years
> Bright shining as the sun,
> We've no less days to sing God's praise
> Than when we first begun.[4]

When we are there, we will be glad all the rest of our endless days, and unanswered prayer and suffering will be put into the glow of eternal blessing. Praise will never reach an end. But Moses' psalm reaches an end with a cry.

> May your deeds be shown to your servants,
>   your splendor to their children.
> May the favor of the Lord our God rest on us;
>   establish the work of our hands for us—
>   yes, establish the work of our hands. (Psalm 90:16-17)

Moses, God's godly servant, wants all of God's servants and their children to witness God's majestic work on earth. He desires God's favor in order that "the work of our hands" will be established. The work of our hands can be confirmed by the favor and loving kindness of the everlasting God.

The work of my hands without God's confirmation and favor are but the work of the flesh, not the gift of the Spirit. But through it all, even while eating dust and standing against the winds of decline, my good work and Becky's good work are confirmed by the everlasting God, who is terrible in his judgments, but rich in his mercy.

When I look at Becky's face, happy or sad, I see what has been taken away, and I see what no earthly cure can touch. But I know that God's favor has not been taken away from his child, that her awareness and intelligence will be restored. But we are still walking through twilight and into a night when no one can work. And God is working still.

Interlude

THE RED BOOK

BECKY MADE THE MOST of her opportunities, especially in writing and editing. She did not waste time and never forgot the kingdom of God and its imperatives. She rightly deemed her writing and editing as her strong points and her major contributions to the world. While talented in music, it would not be her ruling passion and impetus for meaning.

Beginning in 2000 she began a four-year project to coedit a large and ambitious book on women's contributions to the church and society. Her contribution was philosophically rich and, I think, irrefutable. Over four long years Becky wrote and edited the work of over a dozen writers. But that burdensome gestation gave birth to *Discovering Biblical Equality* in 2004.

Twelve years later Becky walked slowly and uncertainly into my basement library and study. Her hands were raised to waist level and were shaking a bit. She grasped at the air to grab words that eluded her. Becky's face was concerned and she looked down. This has become her pathetic pose for communicating. She stammered, "Jane [her caregiver for the weekend] wants the red book." I said, "You mean the book that Jane uses to record her work?" "No," she replied in frustration. "The most important book." I discerned that she meant one of the books she wrote. I stood up and pulled down her first book from my shelf, *Women Caught in the Conflict*. "Is it this one?" "No," she huffed. Then I picked out *Discovering Biblical Equality* and showed it to her. "That one," she said with some relief. I replied, "So that is the most important book of all?" She laughed. She still can laugh at her own misspeaking—for now.

She took it upstairs to give to Jane, but came back down quickly after. "She wants . . . She wants . . ." I figured out that Jane wanted a signed copy, but knew Becky could not write her autograph. "Do you want me to write in it for you?" I asked. "Yes." Jane had put a sticky note on the front of the book that explained what she wanted to have written in the book: "July 17, 2016. To Jane, from Becky Groothuis." This whole operation was a bit confusing to Becky, so I explained what I did. She took her vicariously autographed book up to her kind caregiver.

This woman, once sparkling with intelligence and humor; this woman who wrote two influential books; this woman who coedited a standard work on gender; this woman, my wife, who edited my ten books up until *Philosophy in Seven Sentences*; this woman, Becky, barely had the wherewithal to give her book away. What a miserable reversal! I wondered, *Is this all futility with a thin dusting of meaning, or is it meaning with a thin dusting of futility?* Since *Discovering Biblical Equality* is a thick academic book, the odds of Jane reading much of it are slim. And yet the book has objective worth that is now thrust from our home out into the larger world. It is a gift given and received.

You and I and Becky are "returning to dust," in the words of Psalm 90, each in our own fallen way. We have our own *unknown* timetable. Becky's brain is dusting away before mine. As Becky numbered her days, God established "the works of her hands." That work of study, editing, and writing is being handed down to others.

Becky found much meaning and some joy in her writing. That is long past and will not return. She still finds some joy in giving away her books. But still, Becky can neither sign her name nor remember the title of her book. I taste the bitter dust and cannot spit it out.

> My mouth is dried up like a potsherd,
> > and my tongue sticks to the roof of my mouth;
> > you lay me in the dust of death. (Psalm 22:15)

Ten

LAMENTING
IN THE CLASSROOM

TEACHING DEMANDS MENTAL CLARITY AND DEXTERITY. Becky has lost this. I have not and, please God, must not lose it, because I am a professional teacher and her primary caregiver, as well as her legal guardian and her conservator. Although my aging brain does not perform as it did ten years ago, thus far I can still teach, preach, and write with some facility. No one (that I know of) is suggesting an early retirement. Yet the weight of Becky's illness can unnerve me and compromise my professional abilities and even my teaching.

Halfway through a recent semester, I was put on paid leave by my academic dean for self-care and to organize the chaos that my life had become because of Becky's multifaceted needs. The seminary's dean is both an able administrator and a pastoral man. My first feeling when put on leave was relief, since I had been walking near the edge of the abyss for some time. My second feeling was guilt. I let down my students. My superior quickly redirected me from regret to restoration. That week I told my students of his kind and necessary edict. Some looked disappointed (as was I), but none were angry. A few sent kind notes. I was among friends who cared. One student spoke of mental problems that caused him to lose a semester of school and said, "Dr. Groothuis, you don't need to apologize."

But before nearing the breaking point, I had taught for many years while bearing many woes, many of them stemming from Becky's chronic illnesses, such as fibromyalgia and chemical sensitivities. I could not put on a *game face* while teaching. To use another sports phrase, if I had to *play hurt*, I usually looked hurt. I am not the baseball batter who gets hit on the shoulder by a ninety-five-mile-per-hour fastball and doesn't even rub his shoulder. However, I am keen to wisely incorporate my woes into the wealth of knowledge I want to make known to my students. I hope I am not histrionic or bombastic in my teaching. But I am passionate about what I take to be true and significant, and often think of the fire in Jeremiah's bones to speak God's truth.

> But if I say, "I will not mention his word
>   or speak anymore in his name,"
> his word is in my heart like a fire,
>   a fire shut up in my bones.
> I am weary of holding it in;
>   indeed, I cannot. (Jeremiah 20:9)

Teaching as a Christian is no small thing. The tongues of teachers heal and wound, instruct and beguile, encourage and discourage. This is why James warns teachers, "Not many of you should become teachers, my fellow believers, because you know that we who teach will be judged more strictly. We all stumble in many ways. Anyone who is never at fault in what they say is perfect, able to keep their whole body in check" (James 3:1-2; see also Titus 2:7-8).

Tears can silence the tongue. About twenty years ago, while researching *Deceived by the Light*, I researched the suicide of a young woman who had been influenced by new age ideas about death and the afterlife. I met with her parents and read her suicide note, of which I was given a copy. When I mentioned this in class, I had to stop talking, shed a few tears, and regain my composure. I soon did. Another time, while defending women's abilities to serve God in every way open to a man, I insisted that the church should not disqualify half of its people from using their God-given gifts. I then said that it is bad enough when illness robs someone of ministry, and mentioned my wife. Again, I was quiet and could not talk, fighting back tears (as men usually do in public). Several students prayed for me right then during this awkward time. This was not scripted, and I did not intend for it to have any rhetorical power to support Becky and my position on gender equality.

Now there is a heavier weight to shoulder. I still cannot put on my game face and leave my life's struggles completely out of the classroom (or out of my other writing). But the classroom offers me no wailing wall. So, then, how can my suffering be nobly born before students, none of whom are either my pastor or my therapist? Let me begin with an anecdote from a guest lecture I gave at a secular school.

Nearing the end of my lecture on comparative religion, I shifted subjects. I was speaking on the philosophical problem of evil: How can God be all-good and all-powerful when there is so much suffering in the world? After a brief overview of this issue, I moved from the conceptual to the existential by speaking of my experience with suffering. I said, "My wife has dementia." All eyes—except one set, which was closed—were on me; the fidgeting stopped, and the class was hanging on my words. All teachers savor these moments. Then, I briefly described Becky's condition.

I am wary of emotional promiscuity, but I am learning to graft my sad story into my teaching. In this, I have an authoritative model. When writing of the inhumanity of the German concentration camps, Viktor Frankl was hesitant to be named as author because of "his fear of exhibitionism." Yet *Man's Search for Meaning* became a classic of the twentieth century. That man, a young Jewish psychiatrist, had to speak his name so the tale could be told aright. He was there. I am no Viktor Frankl, but my students seem to benefit by reflecting on suffering through the lens of my lament.

Although I have written about the meaning of suffering and lament, I cannot ignore my obstinate companion when I teach. The classroom—which I strive to make a sanctuary for knowledge—is where I am fully alive, intellectually and emotionally. God has called me to be there. I improvise within the atmosphere of text, teacher, and student. But what does my autobiography have to do with it? It helps that nothing happening in my life is very far from my vocation as a professor. I teach on the problem of evil and I live through the reality of suffering. But we need to be wary of *oversharing* our grief, as my students say. Given all the ego effusions on Facebook, that is easy to do. What should I say and when?

Vernon Grounds, one of my mentors and a longtime professor at my institution, Denver Seminary, said, "When you reveal the viscera in the classroom, you should only go so far." The podium is neither the pastor's study nor the confessional. Both applause lines and tearjerkers should be avoided. Our candor is best shared in measured doses, lest we embarrass our students and ourselves. And yet I teach full-time at a theological institution. We are not merely giving information but investing in our students, many of whom want to hear our stories—and even become a part of them.

By teaching in the first person about our suffering in light of our subjects, teachers may enliven their discourse. (Some very abstract subjects may not benefit from these disclosures, however, such as symbolic logic.) Teachers participate in it rather than only talk about it. This has been my experience in teaching about suffering in the context of lament.

Suffering well before our students also paves avenues for empathic knowledge. Philosophers often define knowledge as justified true belief. But there is another dimension to how humans receive reality. To empathize is to put oneself into the inner world of another. We try to simulate their being in the world. This has epistemic as well as therapeutic benefits. It belongs in both the counseling office and the classroom.

In my courses, I may explain Frankl's theory of suffering by quoting from his books, rephrasing his ideas, discussing them with students, and testing them. Through this, my students gain knowledge. When I add that Frankl's ideas kept me going when I visited my wife in a psychiatric unit, another layer of knowing emerges. Frankl's psychological theory, his story of suffering, and my experience meet in agreement and win a deeper hearing. When I tell my class that I had to "smelt meaning out of suffering" while aspiring to be "worthy of my suffering" (a phrase Frankl drew from Dostoevsky), students begin to empathize with me and learn more from Frankl. They may encounter ideas from the inside out through their emotional perception and imagination.

Seeing through tears may be the truest seeing of all—at least on this side of paradise. So there is no need to ban suffering from pedagogy. I cannot. By suffering well with students, teachers can breathe new knowledge into their classrooms and so curate a community of intellectual achievement and emotional involvement.

Through the suffering of Becky's illness, I may more easily and deeply enter into the suffering of my students. Jesus wept before some of his most profound teaching about death, faith, and the afterlife (John 11:35). We may weep—literally or metaphorically—before our students also.

Eleven

LAMENTING ONLINE

About seven years ago, Becky's best friend set up a Facebook page for her. Sharon wanted a quick way for Becky to stay current with a small circle of friends, most of whom live in another state. Becky appreciated the sentiment but never took it seriously. She eventually asked me to delete it. This was before dementia. Facebook simply did not suit her, although she was still using email. Today, I find few in that company—the Facebook aliens. I am not one of them.

The Internet is colonizing our culture, our commerce, and our souls. Its insinuations and seductions are nearly irresistible. We are told, and tell others, "Go to Google," "check the wiki," and "send a selfie." Now we grieve online. I am not exempt. Facebook is my place for cybergrieving. After a love-hate relationship for several years, Facebook is a firm part of my life. Being an author and speaker, I attract—and often later repel—many "friends" and hover around the maximum friend count for a personal page.

Facebook is more than a tool. It is a way of life, which can be engaged wisely or stupidly. I have done both. I won't give you my full philosophy of Facebook. Rather, let me ponder how Facebook accompanies me in my walk through twilight. The outline for my chapter "The Year of Learning Things I Did Not Want to Know" was first published on Facebook. Of course, I use Facebook for other things, such as social commentary, theology, philosophy, apologetics, humor, and more.

I dare not use Facebook as a substitute for being with friends face to face or talking to them on the phone. Handwritten cards add depth to written communication that is alien to Facebook. Church participation cannot be transposed into cyberspace, although a benighted technophile invented "Saint Pixels" for that purpose some years ago. I need to see and hear and perhaps hug my friends to give and receive solace in my suffering. However, since Facebook reaches so many so quickly, it can be used as a letter, an editorial, a cry for help, a confessional, and a call to prayer.

Denizens of Facebook inform everyone about everything they deem interesting and shareable. You have to filter out and skip over so much cyberstuff to not capsize in the data. I try to not muck up people's screens with trivia or needless emotive effusions. I often fail. However, I can send virtual letters to thousands of people at once. Given the unnerved life I have been living, letting people know of my distress can solicit advice (good and bad), consolation (wise and foolish), and exhortation (proper and improper). These responses are generally helpful to me.

As an inveterate and incorrigible writer, I use Facebook to write short essays on many things, but often about my walk through dementia with Becky. I may describe a scene from our life or editorialize about how Becky's doctors treat her. Somehow, writing about it gives a perspective that lessens the pain and frustration. Readers' responses can be heartening, trivial, or outrageous. But you learn to expect that on Facebook. You can *unfriend* or *block* someone if needed. My essays may be widely shared and commented on. Reporting my pain may lessen others' pain.

When feeling desolate and alone, my posts may be cries for help. Or perhaps they are cries I simply want someone to read. I know that my writing of my distress has helped others give words to their sighs, moans, and cries. Sometimes it is good to know that someone feels the same. My experiences may take the form of unsophisticated poems, which I usually write quickly and do not save. I can also post too much and expose my vulnerabilities unwisely. There are hungry piranhas out there, and I have bite marks to prove it. But the kind souls outnumber the mean fish, thank God.

I have, for good or ill, chosen to lament publicly, to give words to my pain in a public forum. I posted this after an agonizing event.

There are moments when I wonder if the entire history of the universe is worth watching my wife strain for words, her body shaking, wishing she were dead, saying, "Why can't I kill myself?" I am on the bleeding hook to try to find the word, the object. I try elimination: "Is it in the bathroom? Is it a physical object?" Then, I hit on it (again): "Is it your mouth guard?" "Yes!" I soon exhaust every option and cannot find it. I tell Becky, "I cannot find it. We have to wait until tomorrow." She sits there, head in hands while Sunny stares at her, and God remains silent.

The kind souls may post something on my page for the public to read or send me private messages. In a few cases, I have found faithful friends through Facebook. One dear soul, who will likely read these words, volunteered to edit some of my writing since she learned on Facebook that my wife can no longer edit. Her work has been invaluable to me, and, amazingly, her taste in editing is similar to Becky's. Like Becky, she makes my writing better. Like Becky, she does not charge either! A South African friend from Facebook responds quickly—given the time change—to my cries of desolation and also keeps me fed with funny animal videos and Scriptures. I could go on.

Confession is sometimes apropos on Facebook. Perhaps I have failed in my caregiving. I may admit that, warn others not to do the same, and ask for prayer or advice. I may need to apologize for something I posted on Facebook! I confess my sins corporately at my church and hear the words of pardon. Facebook will never take that place, of course. But it may be a place for setting a few things right and breaking down a few walls.

Whatever else the Internet may be, it is a place to solicit and receive prayer. I often post short prayer requests about taking Becky to the doctor or needing to make a crucial decision about her care. In short order, I receive messages from those who pray. This is heartening. In some cases, I can barely pray. The body of Christ needs to step in and lift my weak arms. I tend to be like the apostle Paul (at least in this way) in that I am not shy about asking for prayer: "Devote yourselves to prayer, being watchful and thankful. And pray for us, too, that God may open a door for our message, so that we may proclaim the mystery of Christ, for which I am in chains. Pray that I may proclaim it clearly, as I should" (Colossians 4:2-4). I then often report on the events people prayed for. I try to pray and encourage others too. The significance of wise prayer cannot be overestimated.

As Marshall McLuhan said, "the medium is the message." Facebook shapes how we communicate; it is not a neutral medium. While we set our controls, we do not control its structure. However, I have known it as one meaningful medium for mourning. Becky did not and now cannot. But I may receive some consolation and wisdom from Facebook that I can apply to Becky's ills. For that, I am grateful.

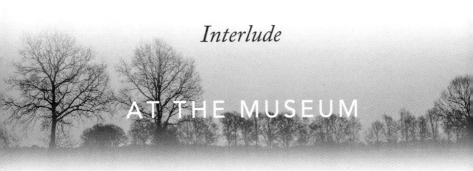

Interlude

AT THE MUSEUM

WHEN YOU CARE FOR SOMEONE WITH DEMENTIA, you try to find activities for the one who is no longer active in the old ways. In our case, most of these fail.

The Denver Art Museum offers activities crafted for those who can no longer act as they did because they can no longer think as they did. The mentally impoverished do not cease to act and crave activities—as long as they can still engage in some goal-directed physical actions. But their actions often lack agency, focused efforts to accomplish something. I see this in Becky often. It is both pathetic and grating, a mixture of sorrow and annoyance. Perhaps, I think, this coordinated art activity, planned by therapists and artists, might help. So, I finally scheduled it.

The event was billed as combining artistic appreciation with music. I scoped and scouted it out as best I could, knowing Becky's condition and unique personality traits. We found our way to the waiting area. No one was alone, of course. As I looked around, it was easy to judge which one in each couple was suffering from dementia. I'm sure others could do the same with Becky and me.

We walked toward the exhibit. The docent was a kind and knowledgeable soul, who made comments about a very large painting depicting a scene filled with all kinds of people. She pointed to people in the painting, asked questions, and elicited responses. She was trying to not talk down to anyone, but she of course failed. It felt awkward. But most of the couples seemed to enjoy it.

Then it got very creative—and terrible for Becky. A number of musicians had been enlisted to play music related to different parts of the painting. They first each demonstrated what their instruments sounded like, something not needed in any other setting. The group was then divided into a number of sections, each of which was given representation of one part of the painting. The group was asked to compose music for each section by working directly with the violinist or horn player. Most warmed to this proposal. Perhaps a low-key bonhomie would even break out (although I felt a gathering dread). It was sheer genius—and sheer distress for Becky.

Those in our group loved it, particularly a talkative man suffering from neither dementia nor self-restraint. He made no reference to his wife or tried to include her in the conversation. She sat there in contented oblivion.

Becky was neither oblivious nor contented, but agitated. She is no extrovert, and strangers are not her forte, especially now. Worse yet, since she is sensitive to sharp sounds and is particular about music, the breakout was not only confusing but irritating. I was helpless again. I excused Becky and myself from the group, again feeling that little in life worked well anymore.

Once we escaped the creative chaos, I walked Becky around a quiet part of the museum where we discussed paintings. Neither of us had much to say, but we were doing something together and, for once, enjoying the environment.

Not long after, we left. I have not had the pluck to attend another made-for-dementia-people art event, although their email solicitations come every week. Perhaps some would be good for Becky. But I don't have the energy to risk another failure. Each email triggers a bad memory. I suppose I should mark them as spam.

Twelve

TECHNOLOGY FREE

Becky and I were usually late adopters of technologies. We were so consumed by reading and writing that we did not invest time to climb the steep learning curve of these new gismos. Yet our writing demanded it as we upgraded our computers and came to terms with the Internet (which *Time* named "Man of the Year" in 1995). At the height of her powers, Becky was using email, mostly for editorial work, using our old landline, and talking on a small, simple cell phone. She started—but soon abandoned—a blog on gender matters, which was well-conceived and well-received. She never went in for chatrooms (good idea) or computer games, and did little to no research online. She was *bookish*. But even her Spartan use of technology began to diminish. She would soon become a technological orphan.

Writing and posting her essays on the blog became bothersome for Becky. Saving and extracting files baffled her. Emails, once so simple, became troublesome. Not knowing the cause of this confusion, I tried to help. I could usually do for Becky what she wanted to do, but I could not teach her how to do it herself. I bought her a new computer that promised to simplify everything. It didn't. She tried and failed to use it. It sat for months. I ended up taking it to my office and then giving it away. As her world was getting thornier and more mystifying, more things were siphoned out of it. What was wrong? We thought it was a symptom of fibromyalgia—fibro-fog. That guess was too optimistic. The truth was, as it often is, far worse.

Becky then began to tussle with her cell phone. She could not make it work. I could not explain it to her. But we still had our reliably simple and pedestrian landline, with its large buttons and long history of use. Now even the landline has been thrown into the same pit as the cell phone, email, and computer. A pen or pencil is beyond her. For about a year Becky could call me using autodial. How often I have remembered the lament of the Preacher: "So I hated life, because the work that is done under the sun was grievous to me. All of it is meaningless, a chasing after the wind" (Ecclesiastes 2:17).

All my efforts—fumbling though they were—to compensate for Becky's losses would at best succeed but for a short time, after which they became obsolete, powerless before the demands of an imperious and implacable enemy called dementia.

All our efforts to compensate for Becky's loss of technological skills are over. Again, I heed the Preacher, my old friend. There is "a time to search and a time to give up, / a time to keep and a time to throw away" (Ecclesiastes 3:6). Any communication is hard won. For now, Becky's understanding exceeds her ability to be understood. Her understanding will erode further, spiraling down into nothing. What she cannot say, she can recognize as her thought when I find the words for her. (This new and necessary ritual of debility is wearisome for both of us, even when we find the words.) These omissions and subtractions in Becky's life spur me to consider a life free of computers and phones of all kinds. Becky had no choice but to opt out, and her extraction from technology often amplifies the ache of her unsolicited solitude.

Having been exiled from most media, Becky is ignorant of current events. This has its advantages, since all contemporary issues are temporary issues when lined up against eternity. Yes, they all have significance in God's economy, and we should serve God and others wherever we can. Yet there is weariness in it and history moves in patterns.

> All things are wearisome,
>> more than one can say.
> The eye never has enough of seeing,
>> nor the ear its fill of hearing.
> What has been will be again,
>> what has been done will be done again;
>> there is nothing new under the sun. (Ecclesiastes 1:8-9)

Moreover, our overexposure to the world's woes can incapacitate us and render us unfit to attend to what is at hand. I sometimes say to Becky, "It is a good thing you don't know much about the external world," and she laughs. But I sometimes relate terrorist attacks and police shootings. She once looked sad and contemplative, and looked at me with big eyes, saying, "What can we do?" "Not much," said I, "but we can pray. I can write about it all and try to bring in truth."

In another way, Becky must use technologies hitherto unneeded. Since she has bouts of sundowner's syndrome, we installed a monitor in her room, so we can help her get back to bed if she wakes up and starts pacing. Eventually, I may have the police set her up with a tracking device in case she wonders off into a dangerous world. As Becky loses her temporal and navigation skills, these technologies will alert us to her actions. The device will not help orient Becky, but it can help us find her.

Becky must limit the channels for giving and receiving information. Her disability demands it, but this sad compensation illustrates a larger principle, applicable to anyone but lost to most: *We are wise to adjust intake to ability*. Put more strongly: we *should* adjust input to ability. What does this mean?

Just as some people have eyes bigger than their stomachs (I am not among them), many of us *ingest* more information than we can *digest*. If so, we are poor stewards of our sensory system. One hundred years ago in the West, information came through only a few media: books, magazines, telegrams, telephones, and radio. The last three media were rare and reached a small percentage of folks. Surely a person can be scatterbrained at any time in history (as a few of my students testify), but in 1917, information moved slowly and was far more scarce than today. Consequently, people were less likely to ingest more than they could digest. The explosion of information technology and the resulting habit of multitasking, skimming, and surfing has ended all that. Americans are well-informed, but all-too-often they are well-informed ignoramuses, as so many polls and man-on-the-street interviews indicate. We should, rather, seek *knowledge* and *wisdom*. Knowledge shifts through information to find truth. Wisdom takes truth and brings it into life with virtue.

Cutting back is essential to going deep. There is a time to skim and a time to *stop and think*. One cannot water ski and deep sea dive at the same time. The great books, for example, require great concentration. Classics require repeated reading. I have poured over C. S. Lewis's *The Abolition of Man*—not a simple book—about ten times over forty years, always reading it in a quiet and solitary place.

Unitasking is often more important than multitasking. The same goes for relationships.

Becky cannot multitask; she can barely unitask. Our conversations demand all of our attention as we hunt down elusive words. (I admit that when Becky interrupts my reading or writing, I am reluctant to do this. I need to repent once again.) Communication technologies have reduced and compromised face-to-face interactions. How can we be *present* with another creature made in God's image when we are *absent*, somewhere else on our smartphone? That is dumb and rude. Is not deep communion with another soul more important than data transfer?

> How good and pleasant it is
>   when God's people live together in unity!
> It is like precious oil poured on the head,
>   running down on the beard,
> running down on Aaron's beard,
>   down on the collar of his robe.
> It is as if the dew of Hermon
>   were falling on Mount Zion.
> For there the LORD bestows his blessing,
>   even life forevermore. (Psalm 133:1-3)

At the end of the apostle John's short letter to "the lady chosen by God and to her children, whom I love in the truth" (2 John 1:1), he writes, "I have much to write to you, but I do not want to use paper and ink. Instead, I hope to visit you and talk with you face to face, so that our joy may be complete" (2 John 1:12; see also 3 John 1:13-14).

My wife can assimilate little information. Her reality is constricting. Her captivity to her disease makes her freer and freer of technology. This simplifies and saddens her life. But even in her decline, she is teaching me—a supposed philosopher of technology— more about personal presence, simplicity, and focus. Becky needs the *unmediated presence* of caring people. We all do.

Thirteen

LEARNING TO LIE
TO MY WIFE
(AS LITTLE AS POSSIBLE)

Dogs must not eat chocolate. It can kill them. We love our dog, Sunny. Sunny, our live-in counselor, is sensitive to our moods. He cares, and he loves to have as much fun as possible. But Sunny must not eat chocolate. Since he does not know this, we must keep chocolate from him. The stakes are high. A dead Sunny would triple our misery.

Our caregiver and I worry that Becky will accidently leave out chocolate, which Sunny will consume at dog speed without any compunction or worry. In a normal household, normal measures are taken. Everyone stays mindful of where chocolate should be. This is not a normal household. Different measures must be taken.

If Sunny eats chocolate and we catch him, we could take him to the veterinarian, who would pump out his stomach. He would likely be fine. Or a little chocolate may not hurt him much. However, these explanations are too complicated for Becky. We tell her this: "Chocolate will kill Sunny." *This categorical* statement is, strictly speaking, false. As a philosopher and as a Christian, I try not to think or speak falsehoods. Indeed, I wrote a book called *Truth Decay*, which tried to prevent it.

However, not every falsehood is a lie. Liars intend to deceive by what they say or do. Say your watch is broken. If you innocently report to a friend that it is 5:30 p.m. when it is 4:30 p.m., this is not a lie. It is a mistake. Lies require one person's intention to deceive someone else about a state of affairs. For example, some volunteers for World War II lied about their age in order to join the military. The cause was noble, but the statements about age were false. A false statement fails to match reality, and reality is never beholden to our beliefs. Truth stands independent of our whims or wishes.

But the statement "Chocolate will kill Sunny" is not an accidental falsehood. I intended to say something that was false. It is a lie, but one not far from the outskirts of truth. "Chocolate will kill Sunny" could be understood as hyperbole, but Becky would not understand it that way. So, it remains a lie. I own it.

This is but one example of prevarication in our household. I wager I can defend lying in these kinds of cases, although the overwhelming majority of lies are morally wrong. But a person with a malfunctioning mind cannot let in the truth like those who are *in their right mind*. Dementia wrongs the mind, violates its integrity, mercilessly attacking it cell by cell. Faculties fade until they are lost. This erosion of *the right mind* tears down and torches the faculties needed to know reality. The brain no longer works properly. Put differently, when a person is mentally compromised, they may not be able to understand the truth we want to tell. Consequently, the words spoken by the right-minded often have no meaning or are misunderstood. One of the features that makes most lies wrong is that they intend to *deceive someone who could have understood the truth*.

If I say to a friend in June 2016, "I am forty-six years old," that statement is false. Accordingly, I am lying to someone who could have understood the true statement, "I am fifty-nine years old." Such a lie is, all things being equal, unjustified.

My mother was suffering from an infection (which eventually killed her) and some dementia in Providence Hospital in Anchorage, Alaska. When I visited, she asked me, "Does my mother know I am in the hospital?" I hesitated a moment and said, "I think so." Nina Cominetto could not have heard a word about her daughter's condition (at least through the normal means) because she passed away in 1985. But then telling my ailing mother that her mother was long dead would have been cruel. She would reexperience her mother's death. Keeping silent would be less cruel, but hurtful as well. This lie was based on what my mother could understand and what was in her best interest, given her abnormal state. As I think back on it now, I should have said categorically, "Yes, she does know, Mom."

The illustration makes a simple argument: whether we lie or tell the truth is sometimes dependent on the state (in this case, mental ability) of the person we address in light of their context. But I am not arguing that we must always shield hard truths from the sick. C. S. Lewis has senior demon Wormwood say in *The Screwtape Letters*:

> How much better for us if all humans died in costly nursing homes amid doctors who lie, nurses who lie, friends who lie, as we have trained them, promising life to the dying, encouraging the belief that sickness excuses every indulgence, and even, if our workers know their job, withholding all suggestion of a priest lest it should betray to the sick man his true condition![1]

To tell a person who can understand his condition that he will recover when he has an untreatable and deadly disease is inexcusable.

It is a lie for a bad purpose to shield someone from a harsh reality they need to know.

Becky and I have trusted each other and have tried to tell each other the truth throughout our marriage. My father was honest to a fault, and I have tried to be as well. However, even as I can justify some lies, given Becky's abnormal condition, they still feel wrong. I do not fear being found out, since Becky cannot. I fear deadening my conscience. The best I can do is to justify lying in extraordinary situations. The prostitute Rahab lied to the authorities of her day in order to protect the two Jewish spies she was hiding (Joshua 2). She is listed as a hero of the faith: "By faith the prostitute Rahab, because she welcomed the spies, was not killed with those who were disobedient" (Hebrews 11:31).

I dare not twist truth for my benefit. But I am not; I am lying to benefit my wife. Although I won't argue it here, the biblical command to "not give false testimony" (Exodus 20:16) does not apply to all lies but rather to cases of using falsehood to hurt other persons, as in a court of law.

Further, one may lie without being a liar by character. As Augustine said, "There is a distinction between a person who tells a lie and a liar. The former is one who tells a lie unwillingly, while the liar loves to lie and passes his time in the joy of lying. . . . The latter takes delight in lying, rejoicing in the falsehood itself."[2] We should earnestly try to never lie, considering exhortations such as this: "Do not lie to each other, since you have taken off your old self with its practices" (Colossians 3:9).

Therapeutic lying is a term some use for telling untruths to those who would be hurt by a truth they could not understand. But there is nothing *therapeutic* about it. It does not make the situation better; it merely keeps it from getting worse for everyone. I will simply call it a *justified lie*. My argument is meant to help in agonizing situations, not to incite a soul to sin by lying to promote or protect oneself. Adam and Eve's fall into sin is the engine of all lies, both sinful and justified (but only in this fallen world). In the world to come, truth will permeate all people, to either their glory or their condemnation. For now, a few lies take a few ounces off the tonnage on Becky's and my backs. Of course, we aspire to fully believe Jesus and thus have no real burden.

> Come to me, all you who are weary and burdened, and I will give you rest. Take my yoke upon you and learn from me, for I am gentle and humble in heart, and you will find rest for your souls. (Matthew 11:28-29)

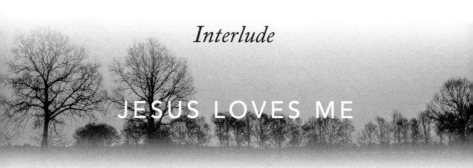

Interlude

JESUS LOVES ME

---

*I pray that the eyes of your heart may
be enlightened in order that you may
know the hope to which he has
called you, the riches of his glorious
inheritance in his holy people.*

EPHESIANS 1:18

I PULLED THE CAR into the garage after a Bible study with some
young friends. Since the meeting went longer than I expected, I
needed to get home and stay home instead of taking a bicycle
ride. Sunny greeted me at the door, as usual. Then I heard
Becky's melodious and distinctive voice, singing a hymn playing
on our stereo. I stopped and listened more closely. She and her
weekend caregiver, who is a Christian, were singing "God
Rescued Me" and then "Rock of Ages." Some of Becky's singing
was wordless. She knew not the words, but she knew the feeling
and the pitch.

When I come home, I usually announce my presence and check
in. But this moment was sacred. I listened in another room for a few
moments, and then slipped downstairs without being noticed. After

writing these words, I went back upstairs to listen from the hallway. They were signing the Gaither's modern standard "He Touched Me." Then they sang

> Jesus loves me this I know,
> For the Bible tells me so.
> Little ones to him belong.
> They are weak, but he is strong.
>
> Yes, Jesus loves me.
> Yes, Jesus loves me.
> Yes, Jesus loves me.
> The Bible tells me so.

I wept. Profundity and simplicity sang through debility. Becky cannot say these words. But she can sing them—and mean them.

Becky and her caregiver were singing and communing with their God. Their eyes were closed. But the eyes of their hearts were not closed. Paul's prayer for his beloved Ephesians spilled over and was answered for his sisters in Christ two thousand years later. Surely Becky one day will experience in fullness "the riches of his glorious inheritance in his holy people" (Ephesians 1:18).

Fourteen

GALLOWS HUMOR

HUMANS LAUGH. I think Sunny does too, but not because he picked up on some irony, a twist in the meaning of a word or phrase, or a parody. He laughs for the joy of playing with a toy and when he greets us. He wiggles, stretches, turns in circles, and sneezes. Becky and I laugh too—with Sunny and sometimes even at the heartbreaking realities we face. We don't usually wiggle, stretch, or sneeze, but we do laugh. Dementia is deadly serious. It is no laughing matter. Or is it?

Laugher plays many roles. There is the laugh of ridicule, derision, or sarcasm. There is no happiness there. There is the laugh of nervousness, which can become an unconscious habit, a tick. It is barren of joy. Even God laughs without being happy.

> The wicked plot against the righteous
>   and gnash their teeth at them;
> but the Lord laughs at the wicked,
>   for he knows their day is coming. (Psalm 37:12-13)

God laughs in that he recognizes the absurd futility of any revolt against him. This is a laugh no one should want to hear, and it cannot give God pleasure, lest he be a sadist (Ezekiel 33:11).

Mocking laughter is neither funny nor godly, as the Bible affirms frequently in Proverbs and elsewhere: "The proud and arrogant person—'Mocker' is his name—behaves with insolent fury" (Proverbs 21:24). The mocker is akin to the scoffer:

> Blessed is the one
>> who does not walk in step with the wicked
> or stand in the way that sinners take
>> or sit in the company of mockers. (Psalm 1:1)

A Christian should laugh, but never mock or scoff in the biblical sense of flippant and mean-spirited derision.

Humor may not elicit laughter, but merely a smile or the thought *That was clever*. Contrariwise, a joke or amusing comment may induce paroxysms of mirth. When in college, I for the first time played a cut from a Monty Python record for a friend. It is called "Ann Elk's Theory of the Brontosaurus."[1] At the comedic climax, my friend emitted a short, loud shriek, spun out of his chair, and began undulating on the floor while making whimpering sounds in between gasps for air. This was completely involuntary—and perhaps hazardous. Humor has power.

Philosophers, psychologists, and others puzzle over the nature and causes of humor. Freud, being Freud, thought it a release of unconscious and unpresentable thoughts. Freudian slips may be funny, but we need better counsel on the nature of humor. But I fear humor is like what Augustine said about time in *The Confessions*: I know what it is until I am asked to explain it. Humor is, well, humorous and not serious, lighthearted and not heavyhearted, clever and not stupid. But I have still not defined it. Consider three theories, all which help us understand humor but none of which, taken by itself, explains all of it.[2]

The superiority theory claims that humor trades on putting someone in their place. It is clever ridicule, an insult. Shakespeare was a master at it. Here is a jab at the corpulent: "Thou art no Atlas for so great a weight."[3] Lady Astor, who often jousted with Winston Churchill, said to him, "If you were my husband, I'd poison your tea." Churchill replied, "Madame, if you were my wife, I'd drink it." Ridicule may be funny, but it cannot be humor's essence, since we often laugh without ridicule.

Then there is *the incongruity theory*. Humor finds something in the world that is odd, unexpected, and entertaining. This often involves juxtapositions, surprises, and double meanings. In a Pink Panther film, Peter Sellers sees a small dog in a hotel's lobby. He asks the attendant, "Does your dog bite?" "No" is the reply. The dog then bites Sellers as he tries to pet him. He says, "I thought you said your dog did not bite!" The attendant replies, "That is not my dog."[4] The scene pulls us one way (the expected meaning), then pulls the other way (the unexpected meaning). We laugh.

The relief theory asserts that humor allows pent-up fear to be released in unexpected ways. Before giving an evangelistic sermon, I found myself uncharacteristically overwrought. Just before I was to give my message, two young women performed a lovely interpretive dance. When it was done and I stood behind the pulpit and said, "I was going to dance for you, but after that . . ." I was relieved at once and got a good laugh from the congregation. I then gave a serious message with little humor.

But we laugh at many things. We may laugh at the wrong things.[5] Some laughter is cruel, however clever it may be. One can laughingly ridicule a man in a wheelchair, or make him laugh and help him forget that he is in a wheelchair. Humor is double-edged. It may open our hearts or slam them shut. There is nothing funny about Becky's condition itself. To ridicule it would be sadistic. But humor can find odd angles of vision on even the worst situations and without rancor or ridicule.

Without humor, Becky and I would be far more miserable than we are. Before Becky's decline, we would often engage in spirited repartee, which often required some esoteric ideas. And, yes, we would be quite pleased with ourselves. It was uniquely *our humor*. But we did not keep it to ourselves. Although Becky ventured out less and less as her sickness increased, our times out with others were often animated and amusing. At her prime, Becky's wit was sharp, sophisticated, unsparing, and (usually) good-natured.

Humor is a fine escape for anyone, as long as it isn't unclean, mean, or stupefying. Becky and I can no longer climb into the heights of rarified humor, but we can still laugh. We sometimes escape into humor by watching old *Seinfeld* videos or by watching our canine comedian, Sunny, ebulliently leap high into the air before eating his dog food. We laugh when we see him scamper around the house at top speed simply because he feels like it. This humor removes us from Becky's memory loss, speech loss, happiness loss, and the near loss of faith. It is *other* than all that.

Although she was not diagnosed with dementia at the time, I first began to worry about Becky when she got lost driving home from a haircut. After several hours, we got her home, but I was emotionally battered. I had to give an apologetically oriented sermon the next day. Amazingly, the message went smoothly. I was more humorous than usual. (I hope not too much.) How odd that levity visited my crushed spirit. But even these early signs of Becky's dementia—fearful though they were—could not quench my humor. In the end, joyful laughter must be stronger than tears.

Another kind of humor takes us into our losses, but has no element of ridicule. It is a form of *gallows humor*, which laughs in the face of death and decay, robbing it of some of its grim sobriety.

The online Oxford Dictionary defines it as "Grim and ironical humour in a desperate or hopeless situation."[6]

Since Becky came home from the Senior Behavioral Health unit of Lutheran Medical Center, we have sporadically discussed her time there. We often refer to it as "the funny farm" and the patients as "inmates." This is gallows humor indeed, since being locked into a facility that treats those with serious mental illnesses is grim. Of course, we laugh more about it now than when Becky was an inmate.

Irving Goffman studied mental health asylums (as they were then called), and found them to be "total institutions." There is little choice. Times to eat, sleep, and congregate are determined by others. You cannot come and go as you please. The doors lock against your will.[7] When Becky was first put into the behavioral health unit, my friend Sarah and I visited her. We asked the nurse to unlock the door. As we walked down a long hall and went through the doors, Sarah asked, "Did you hear the guy walking behind us?" I did not. She then told me he was trying to catch up without running. He was an inmate. He was trying to escape.

Given Becky's speech losses, I am usually the one to make these humorous comments about "funny farms" and "inmates." Our closeness over many years gives me a comedic freedom not afforded to others. Becky cannot dish it out as she used to. But she can take it and laugh.

Getting food from the table and into her mouth can be puzzling to Becky. Several times I have seen her eat from a plate that was pushed several inches away from where a plate should be. I look at Becky and then at the plate, and remark in sardonic tones, "Do you think it should be a little closer?" We laugh. She may ponder her spoon and fork, not knowing which to use for a particular helping.

I say something like, "It's a tough decision, isn't it?" We laugh. It can get bizarre, but remains funny. While having breakfast out, Becky dispensed with utensils altogether and began eating her fried potatoes with her fingers, not sensing any impropriety. I noted, "So, you've given up entirely on forks, I see." We laugh. But she laughs first, so I know she is not mimicking me.

After we had dinner one night, I anomalously left a piece of pie with cream on the dining room table and went to my desk to do some paperwork. (Me doing paperwork can be quite humorous in itself.) Becky soon walked to me with that piece of pie, but without a fork. I said, "Where's the fork?" She looked perplexed and said she didn't know where they were. I went with her into the kitchen, opened the utensil drawer, pointed, and said, "Well, there they all are." We both laughed again.

Becky and I enjoyed an early dinner at Olive Garden. We were both in relatively good spirits and laughed at each other. On the way there, I said, "Maybe if you get drunk, you'll come back to normal." She laughed. I said, "It's the Jimi Hendrix principle. He was so weird that one dose of LSD brought him back to normal." We laughed. We also laughed at the idiosyncrasies of her eating. We were laughing together about something utterly serious. This chemistry materializes only in rare settings and relationships.

A couple about our age was seated near us not long after we came in. As we were leaving, I noted that Becky and I had talked and laughed far more than this couple, neither of whom seemed to have mental problems. Their brain chemistry was fine, but perhaps they lacked the comedic and existential chemistry that Becky and I can still delight in.

Becky's humor, while not so fine-grained as it was, remains more intact than most of her other mental functions. While the tears outnumber the smiles, and the quaking of despair is more common than the movement of laughter, Becky's mirth is as yet unbroken. I grab on to what I can, even though I know my grip is loosening.

Fifteen

DOGS, DEMENTIA, AND US

OUR DOG, SUNNY, IS A GOLDENDOODLE, and, I am sure, a gift from God given to comfort and amuse Becky and me in the worst moments of dementia. Therapy dogs (properly certified) were part of the hospital team when Becky stayed at the behavioral health unit for five weeks in 2014. They even have business cards, which their humans obediently hand to anyone interested. Sunny is not officially a therapy dog, but I call him "our best counselor."

For about a year after Becky's release from the hospital, she could take Sunny on a walk by herself. But we put a tag on Sunny that says on one side, "Help. My mother has dementia." On the other is my contact information. After both were brought home in a police car, Becky and Sunny cannot go on walks by themselves.

As much as I love dogs, as a Christian, I am taken aback by what the Bible says about Sunny's species. I try to regulate my loves according to reality, so as to not multiply my vain losses. I need to think this out. Perhaps I am too sentimental.

Dogs are neither popular nor praised in the Bible. Ecclesiastes writes, "a live dog is better off than a dead lion" (Ecclesiastes 9:4). Even a lowly dog trumps a lion, but only if the latter is dead and the former still barks. When he was tussling with Saul, David said to the king: "Against whom has the king of Israel come out? Who are you pursuing?

A dead dog? A flea? May the Lord be our judge and decide between us. May he consider my cause and uphold it; may he vindicate me by delivering me from your hand" (1 Samuel 24:14-15).[1] David, apparently not a dog lover, ranks "man's best friend" with a flea, and recoils at being associated with either pest. Since no one, I take it, has ever had a pet flea, things look grim for the canine clan. In the Bible, calling someone a "dog" meant that they were disreputable or worse.

When a Syrophoenician woman entreated Jesus to heal her demon-possessed daughter, Jesus initially refused to answer her, saying he was sent "only to the lost sheep of the house of Israel." She then cried, "Lord, help me!"

> He replied, "It is not right to take the children's bread and toss it to the dogs." "Yes it is, Lord," she said. "Even the dogs eat the crumbs that fall from their master's table." Then Jesus said to her, "Woman, you have great faith! Your request is granted." And her daughter was healed at that moment. (Matthew 15:26-28)

The nameless woman turned Jesus' reference to dogs to her own benefit. Jesus then commended her faith and answered her wish. However, the reference to a dog's master indicates that some were domesticated and a few were allowed to eat crumbs (as is Sunny).

Yet our dog is a gift of God in our desolation. The thought of separating Becky and Sunny is almost too much for me to think about. I want them together as long as possible.

In 2012 a friend finally convinced us to get a dog. I had long wanted one, having loved them since growing up with Nina, a husky–German shepherd mix. But Becky was allergic to so many things that having a dog seemed like one more difficulty to manage. I pined for a pooch, but had given up.

But our friend, a dog lover and animal trainer, made it easy. She found a breed that was affable, smart, and did not shed—the goldendoodle, which is half golden retriever and half standard poodle. Sarah contacted a top-notch breeder, who had a litter of four pups for us to see on Skype. We beheld an eight-pound pup called Whitey, because of a white streak on his chest. He captured us in a moment. Whitey arrived in a small kennel at Denver International Airport. I thought his name was to be Sonny, after the jazz tenor-sax titan Sonny Rollins. (Becky had refused Trane, for John Coltrane.) But Sunny fit his character better than the name of a jazz musician, so Sunny he was. But I later learned that Sunny had good chops and big ears.

Our friend knew that we needed what a dog had to offer. While Becky had not yet been diagnosed with dementia, we knew she was in decline—depressed, unsettled, and at odds with life. I told my mentor that I envisioned nothing more for my marriage than managing the decline of my wife. We could not be consoled by our children; we had none. We could not be consoled by our parents; they were gone. But Sunny came.

Sentimentality may undermine serious writing about dogs and other pets. Philosophers speak of the *pathetic fallacy*, through which we falsely attribute uniquely human emotions and thoughts to animals, who do not possess them. For example, a dog's muteness beckons us to speak for her: "Bonnie says she doesn't think puppies are fun." This border collie turns up her intelligent and no-nonsense nose in the company of pups. In this case, Bonnie's ventriloquist seems to have gotten it right. But can we be so sure in other cases? Dogs cannot tell us what they are thinking. They can show mannerisms, expressions, and actions, from which we infer their mental and emotional states.

Nevertheless, I find myself saying (as you may, as well), "I wish I were a dog." No sane Israelite would wish that. Dogs today, if not yesterday, seem to have a blissful life—no bills to pay, no buttons to push, no concern, it seems, about death. But I wonder. When my childhood dog, Nina, was badly injured, our friend Floyd carried her eighty-pound body out the door to the veterinarian. As he was about to leave, Nina looked at my mother with such sadness and resignation that my mother remembered it forty years later. Nina died at the vet. My mother cried when she recounted this to me. Since dogs are affected by the fall as well as the rest of creation, their lives are not without distress. But still, their zeal, their being in the moment (like jazz musicians), may inspire jealousy. Essayist and dog lover James Thurber wrote that "Man is troubled by what might be called the Dog Wish, a strange and involved compulsion to be as happy and carefree as a dog."[2]

Another trap for those philosophizing about dogs is egotism. Dogs unconditionally love owners who treat them well. They are quick to forgive (if that is the right word) small offenses.[3] I cannot verify this, but I imagine that Blondie, Adolph Hitler's German shepherd, loved and was obedient to the fuehrer, who cared for his dog far better than he did millions of human beings. When he knew he had lost the war, Hitler brought Blondie to his Berlin bunker, where he killed her, along with his mistress, Eva Braun. He then committed suicide.

It may be that our love for dogs is self-centered. We imagine that they are so discerning to love us as they do. But remember Blondie. With these killjoy caveats in mind, let us return to Sunny and his kin in order to consider their part in walking through twilight.

As a puppy, Sunny elicited laughter and abundant joy in those who saw and played with him. Soon after we picked up the furry bundle at Denver International Airport, a couple about my age came over to see him. The man laughed continuously for about ten minutes simply at seeing the puppy's visage. His wife delighted in showing us the best place to pet his head.

Now, of course, all puppies—and most young animals—are cute. The cuteness in dogs often oozes a charmed balm that assuages suffering and releases joy. What is *cuteness*, though? We know it when we see it, but we also disagree about it. Innocence, prettiness, and attractiveness make up cuteness, as I take it. Living and nonliving things may be cute, both a stuffed animal and a baby bird. Cuteness disarms us, makes us smile and emit cooing sounds. Cuteness observed and misery felt will never coincide. A good lick on the face may console us, even when the hot tears flow, the body heaves in grief, and the last drop of hope seems to dissolve into an ebony ocean of despair.

Dogs are as much a product of culture as they are of nature. God created each thing according to its kind. I take it that "canine" is a *kind* or perhaps a subset of a biblical *kind*. Thus, the essence of dog spans a wide spectrum of critters. The genetics of the species allows for great plasticity. Both a teacup poodle and a Saint Bernard are canines, as is a wolf, their ancestor. This variation is due more to unnatural selection than natural selection. Dogs have been selectively bred for different purposes, as have horses and many other animals. They have been domesticated, unlike a bear or an octopus.[4]

We domesticate animals because we are made in God's image and likeness (Genesis 1:26). It is of our essence to cultivate and develop creation, inanimate and animate, through our God-given gifts under God's authority and according to his revelation. All animals have value as God's creatures, since God endorsed his prehuman creation as *good* (Genesis 1). Animals may be good gifts to people, and people may be good gifts to animals. "The righteous care for the needs of their animals, / but the kindest acts of the wicked are cruel" (Proverbs 12:10).

Without developing a whole theology of animals, I note several items about dogs per se. First, while dogs have a nature, that nature is plastic, both genetically and existentially. A dog left to roam ancient Palestine and fend for itself among other similarly disadvantaged dogs is not likely to be cuddly. Such a dog may even be dangerous. It would not have been clean. The biblical dog lived before dog-training classes, veterinarians, and the Humane Society. This seems to explain the slams on dogs in the Bible. Serpents get even worse press, of course, but I won't defend them.

Second, the breeding of dogs partly fulfills God's call on us to develop and cultivate the earth (Genesis 1:26; Psalm 8:4-8). Dogs were domesticated long ago and bred from wolves to assist humans in hunting (poodles), tracking (bloodhounds), herding (border collies), protection (bullmastiff), conveyance (sled dogs, such as huskies), and much else. Dogs today are usually for human comfort and companionship. My first dog, Nina, was part husky, but she was no sled dog. She was domesticated and not used for conveyance, as some of her cousins still are. Sunny is a *comfort dog* alone and extraordinaire.

Third, James tells us to recognize the benevolence of God in salvation and in all else. Dogs may be one aspect of this kindness.

Don't be deceived, my dear brothers and sisters. Every good and perfect gift is from above, coming down from the Father of the heavenly lights, who does not change like shifting shadows. He chose to give us birth through the word of truth, that we might be a kind of first fruits of all he created. (James 1:16-18)

A good dog is a gift, which, at its doggy best, dimly mirrors some qualities of its Maker, particularly unconditional love. Sunny is quick to forgive, senses our moods astutely, and comforts us aggressively when we despair. Sunny's manifest love eases the pain.

This love is an analog of God's character. Sunny at his best is also an incentive for me to be more loving, sensitive, and affectionate in my care of Becky. Sunny trusts unconditionally, which mirrors what our trust of God should be. Martin Luther owned a "dog named Tölpel (which was apparently a synonym for 'Dummkopf')." Luther saw in his dog a quality he wanted to possess. "Oh, if I could only pray the way this dog watches the meat! All his thoughts are concentrated on the piece of meat. Otherwise he has no thought, wish, or hope."[5]

In their earnestness and openness, dogs can also teach us to enjoy the moment deeply and not worry about tomorrow (although Sunny gets a bit worried at the vet). John Homans puts it well:

> This state of being-in-the-moment is what's so compelling about dogs. It's hard for a human to get to it. Even in the most difficult times, dogs are cheerful and ready for experience. A dog can't figure out that it's being measured for its grave. The three-legged chow that walks on my street every day doesn't know the number three or have any sense that anything is wrong with her at all. . . . It's not that a dog accepts the cards it's been dealt; it's not aware that there are cards.[6]

Becky and I are aware of the cards we have been dealt, but we also are aware of our dog and join him in the cheerful moments. During this canine respite, we are not worrying about the loss of memory and speech; we are not worrying about getting along with the caregivers; nor are we anguishing over Becky's needs as she worsens.

Of course, some souls will rule out dogs as companions and comfort, either because of allergies or because of their temperament as extreme feline lovers. Nevertheless, dogs are a tonic for despair for many of us—and perhaps even a foretaste of the frolic and fun in the world to come.[7]

Sixteen

MISS BECKY AND A WAY OF SPEAKING

Adults usually talk differently to children, but I don't think my parents did. I was raised around adults more than most, since my parents entertained often and I had no brothers or sisters. I remember being bothered at parties when adults would interrupt me. I may have been a child, but I had something to say. I didn't want to be spoken to with a special voice. I could sense when I was talked down to and despised it. In fourth or fifth grade our class watched a film that was below our level. In an annoying sing-song voice, the narrator said something like, "And don't you want to know X?" I said to the teacher afterward, "What if I don't want to know X?" The kids laughed. In other words, "Don't talk down to me. I'll make my own intellectual decisions. So there."

Early on, after Becky was diagnosed, I noticed that people began to speak to her differently. No one is able to penetrate the density that dementia brings. The doors are closing, and, later, nothing will go in or out. Nevertheless, when addressing a woman who had been in Mensa, who wrote two books (and coedited another), and who was more intelligent than I am, people now tend to raise their voice (hearing is not her problem, yet), lapse into sing-song and upward inflection, and refer to her in terms they would never use for any right-minded adult—terms like *hon* or *dear* or other inapt terms of awkward endearment.

Perhaps worse yet, somewhere on this tortuous road into mental oblivion, she earned the title "Miss Becky." Mind you, we are not in Louisiana. When in New Orleans, I was summoned as "Mr. Douglas" in an emergency room. That is their custom. "Miss Becky" is not the custom in Denver or anywhere else Becky and I have lived. I suppose children receive this moniker: "Now, Miss Julie, get ready for bed right now. Then I'll tell you a bedtime story." "Yes, Mommy," says Miss Julie.

Patronizing is the word for it. Becky is still an adult, not a child. She is not *Miss Becky*, blast it. Please, do not condescend. Speak in normal tones, but be prepared to repeat, rephrase, point, and to give up with compassion when you cannot get through. But there is something worse with words.

I have to interpret the world for Becky and help others understand her world. I am a linguistic mediator: from Becky to world and from world to Becky. Doctors, and there are so many we have to see, need to talk to me about Becky's condition, since she cannot report much. The kind ones ask her a question and then look to me if she cannot answer. The insensitive ones talk to me: "Is she eating enough?" This *second person reference*, when voiced in front of the patient, is not merely condescending, it is dehumanizing. She is not invited into a conversation, however grim it may be. She is an entity to be described and (if possible) treated. If a friend comes to my house and asks, "Is Sunny over his rash?" all is well, since Sunny is oblivious. Becky is not. Worse yet is when someone speaks of Becky in the second person, assuming she cannot understand them. Someone said, "She won't wander around, because she is too hungry to leave the table." To someone in their right mind, this would be insulting and wounding. Accordingly, it should not be uttered. We often need to treat those who are not all there as if they were all there. Otherwise we will not retain our respect for the crippled human being in our midst. Just as in teaching, it is better to talk over someone's head than to insult their intelligence.

We are not speaking to a child but to an adult trying to retain her vanishing maturity. Yes, she is childlike, but she is not growing up. She is falling down—inch by inch, day by daunting day. She has lost what she cannot regain. She is not a child. Do not speak to her as if she were.

Then how should we speak? Let me speak for myself. I must interpret and navigate the world for my declining wife more than anyone else. I narrate the obvious to one becoming oblivious to fact. This is tiring. "Let's get out of the car and walk to the museum," I say. Then I take her hand, not so much out of affection but out of necessity. I remember when Becky was attentive to things I was not. She helped me observe and interpret the world (and God). We laughed together over much of it. Occasionally, she still does. As we drive, she points to the clouds over the Rocky Mountains. "Look at those . . ." I have seen clouds a million times, but not *these clouds*. These clouds give my wife delight right now. "Clouds," I say. "Yes." I provide the word for the thought, and it aids appreciation. She once provided better words for my writing when she was my live-in editor.

Narration is often coupled with Becky's need for physical assistance. I ask if she wants a Jacuzzi. I draw the water and tell her I will come back in half an hour to help her out because she lacks both agency and attentiveness. I then assume both faculties and try to do what she cannot do for herself. I am vicarious in ways I never imagined. I stand-in where she falls down. This, makes me a bit like Christ, who did for us what we could never do: atone for our sins, stand in our place, give our short lives meaning, and grant us eternal life. The prophet Isaiah, God's prophet, foretold a sacrifice and substitution unlike any other.

> Surely he took up our pain
>   and bore our suffering,
> yet we considered him punished by God,
>   stricken by him, and afflicted.
> But he was pierced for our transgressions,
>   he was crushed for our iniquities;
> the punishment that brought us peace was on him,
>   and by his wounds we are healed.
> We all, like sheep, have gone astray,
>   each of us has turned to our own way;
> and the LORD has laid on him
>   the iniquity of us all. (Isaiah 53: 4-6; see also 1 Peter 2:24-25)

Jesus, the long-promised Messiah, through his incomparable suffering, took our pain, our suffering, and our punishment, and gave us in their place peace and divine direction. The sheep gain a shepherd. The felons find their pardon. The accused are acquitted. The gospel is fulfilled. And we are commissioned to do the same. As Paul said so simply, "Carry each other's burdens, and in this way you will fulfill the law of Christ" (Galatians 6:2). He also counseled, "We who are strong ought to bear with the failings of the weak and not to please ourselves" (Romans 15:1).

I speak *to* Becky and I speak *for* Becky. People frequently speak in the interrogative mood when someone has the faculties to say yes or no rationally. "Do you want to have a Jacuzzi?" But those with little understanding have little *agency*. An agent has (1) the will to act, (2) the ability to act, and (3) the understanding to act rationally.

We usually do things—or try to do things—for reasons, whether good or bad. I buy yet another book on suffering to further my expertise in misery. (Why did God not choose another soul better equipped?) As an agent, I (1) decide to buy the book, (2) have the ability to buy the book, and (3) have reasons for buying the book.

But when the world recedes, the understanding finds little to work with. This erodes informed volition. I often see Becky milling about, not knowing what to do next—and often not knowing what she has just done. Her brain is losing *executive function*, which, physically speaking, resides in her frontal lobes. Primary progressive aphasia, the name for her plague, is a frontal lobe disease. Executive function requires the ability to:

1. Analyze a task.
2. Plan how to address the task.
3. Organize the steps needed to carry out the task.
4. Develop timelines for completing the task.
5. Adjust or shift the steps, if needed, to complete the task.
6. Complete the task in a timely way.[1]

For the strong one, kind commands should fill this volitional void. "Let's have a Jacuzzi." "Let's go for a walk with Sunny." "Let's go to Olive Garden." "We are going to an art tour." These imperatives are not imperious, since I am not imposing my will on a resistant agent. Rather, I am *substituting* my will for hers in order to assist her in her actions. It is vicarious. I supply the purpose in something I hope (usually in vain) she will find meaningful and enjoyable. I *enjoin* her in light of what eludes her. It is more of an *invitation* (when done well) than an unyielding *command* from the Decalogue. My words direct her and correct her in ways uncommon to our yesterdays. Of course, in my proxy judgments and invitations, I ponder what is in her best interest. Once we tried to discern our best interests together, working as a loving and critical team. And so I lament the loss of our conversations, crackling with her intelligence and clever humor.

A deacon from my Anglican church knows how to speak with Becky. Because Becky does not fare well in my church or in most public gatherings (unlike many dementia victims), Katie, an Anglican deacon, came to our home to serve Communion. She greeted Becky, Sunny, and me with her customary warmth. The three of us talked a bit before receiving the Eucharist. Katie looked into Becky's eyes, listened, and spoke lovingly, without any affectation or artificiality. She knew Becky was not in her right mind, but did not talk down to her because she was not in her right mind.

Dear right-minded and well-meaning people: speak like Katie.

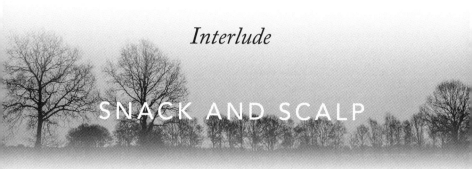

Interlude

SNACK AND SCALP

BECKY CAME DOWN THE STAIRS. I dread these visits, since she will almost always be distressed and want my help. I am usually amendable to assist, but detecting what help she needs is often difficult, unsuccessful, and painful for both of us. Not this time, though.

Smiling, she asked if I wanted to eat a little package of snacks, which are reserved for her in a special place that she (for now) can remember. I agreed (since I never turn down food) with a surprised smile. After I said thank you, she looked pleased, and went upstairs. We were both happy in a simple act of generosity. I made sure Sunny couldn't eat them before I did.

Becky often talks about wanting to do some good now that her writing, editing, and household management skills are gone. I often tell her to pray for me and for other needs. She used to wash my clothes, something she had done since we got married. She resolutely (and wisely) denied my infrequent requests to learn how to wash (and iron). For months, she would wash the same load many times, mix the whites and the colors, and lose myriad socks (which gave the opportunity for me to mismatch them). But when the mistakes crossed a threshold, our caregiver took over. Since her return from the hospital, Becky cleaned my bathroom, something she did seldom before. (I think she had been fearful to scan it.) Once again, her efforts, so well-intended, accomplished little, and left me looking for bathroom items. That too came to an end. Becky had one less way to serve.

Becky will often ask, "What can I do to help?" This repeatedly baffles me. She will offer to rub my scalp, something Sunny and I both enjoy. I accept. The woman who once kept our books, once wrote books, once edited books, once shopped, once cooked (a little)—this woman can offer none of this. She knows this and suffers. I do not so much miss her service but the one who could serve.

But for a few moments, Becky served me with a smile. It was relaxing, as it always is. It wasn't complicated. There was no stammering, stuttering, or frustration. Thank you, Becky.

I keep waiting. Becky keeps waiting. Who knows when we may be surprised by the goodness that punctuates the increasing darkness with scattered light?

Seventeen

WORDS FAIL US

THOSE WITH ALZHEIMER'S can usually speak until close to the end, even if they don't know what they are saying. From the beginning of dementia, Becky, the wordsmith, editor, and writer, has sought words in vain. It has gotten progressively worse and will not get better. Words are failing her and, in a different way, failing me as well.

Before taking Sunny for a grooming, Becky wanted me to go upstairs so she could point at some kind of problem relating to clothes. She could say *clothes*. I did not have time. She did not want to wait, since her leaky memory would not retain it. But it did retain it.

When I returned, we reengaged our foe, *futility*. We went into her bedroom to pursue the problem of clothes. She pointed to her drawers, the words still failing even as other words were nervously repeated. They were not the right words, the absence of which was tormenting her. She took me into her closet. I had no idea what she wanted, so we went back to her drawers. I kept offering possible words—and failing. Words failed her in one way, and they failed me in another. I then tried categories: old clothes or new clothes, casual clothes or dress clothes, underwear of outerwear. "No, no!" she said, her body shaking in unalloyed frustration. *Agonizing* is too mild of a word for this. Words failed me, as they failed her. Words for objects do not (usually) fail me; words for new and terrible emotional states do fail me. Would that I not have to learn this vocabulary of lament! I am at a loss for words. I, the wordsmith, editor, and writer, sought out words in vain.

Through Becky and my fatiguing hunt for a single word, I had to be at once a detective, a counselor, and a saint. I had to fight off anger. God does give me patience, and I needed a supernatural dose. I had to piece together clues to find the meaning. I had to keep Becky calm. All this was not her fault, but she would not let up. I implored her, "You have plenty of clothes and we can talk about it later." "No!" was her reply.

Somehow, the right word, the sequestered word, appeared: *shorts*. She did not have enough shorts. I found most of them in a basket of freshly washed clothes. I handed them to her. But that wasn't enough either, since the shorts (at least the ones I could find) were all casual. She needed better ones. "We will look for better ones later, and buy new ones if we need to." Since frustration had eclipsed consolation, Becky hung her head in despair as I left the room. This verbal futility crushed a day's worth of emotional energy into ten long minutes, and we too were crushed.

Becky and I once lived for finding and savoring the right words, the best sentences, the strongest arguments. This attracted us to each other in 1983. She edited and counseled me through my first book. She was an articulate and humorous speaker with a pleasant voice. Our repartee was rewarding and unreproducible outside of us. That was then. To quote the Beatles, "Yesterday came suddenly." Yesterday comes every day. Becky's loss for words forces me to reflect more on language and its losses. So often she either has nothing to say or can say nothing. Perhaps my own words in this book will serve the Word—Jesus Christ—and those who serve him with words.

Given the fall, none of us speaks or writes perfectly all the time, but some of us strain for perfection. If I misspeak even *once* in a sermon or lecture, it hurts; although, in my dotage, I am mellowing on this, giving myself permission to be human. I cultivate a large vocabulary. During my first year in college, I was surprised and intimidated by all the new words I found in my textbooks. (We were all assigned textbooks in the pre-Internet, primordial past.) I circled them, consulted the *American Heritage Dictionary* my mother gave me before I left for college in 1975 (I still have it), and recorded these new items of knowledge in a black, blank book. I added word to word, page to page, for about twenty years. The blank book had no page numbers, so I added them. I filled up over a hundred pages. I have not counted the number of words, but I know that I repeated some. I often show this to my students to fire their zeal for vocabulary.

I read books on building *word power*. I became scrupulous about finding the proper words and putting them into grammatically impeccable sentences. I read books by language sticklers, curmudgeons who exhorted me to write and speak well. Two books by (amazingly enough) the *television* reporter Edwin Newman taught me to love proper English usage. *Strictly Speaking* and *A Civil Tongue* scolded the lazy tongue and encouraged articulate utterance.[1] In those days, when I watched television (which was so different then), *Firing Line*, with William F. Buckley, was one of my favorite programs. His debonair command of language paired with his indefatigable wit and vast knowledge were awe-inspiring. Television has since ceased to inspire in me any awe, but it *is* awful.

Along the way I developed a theology of writing and speaking. In order to express truth aright, one must develop and employ verbal precision. (And I knew that *verbal*, popular opinion to the contrary, referred to both written and spoken language.) Since God is the source of all truth as the Logos, and since God has revealed himself to us in language (the Bible), and since we must bear intelligent and winsome witness to God's truth, we need to speak and write well. Beneath these noble sentiments was some ego: I prized my own abilities and diligence in mastering English. (I have never mastered another language, to my shame.)

Becky did much the same. She loved and revered language. So when we met, we found instant camaraderie. She often corrected my speaking and writing. I seldom had to correct hers. But all the tools of language—the style guides, dictionaries, thesauruses—do Becky no good now. Her books, her erstwhile friends, now sit in *my* library. In fact, Becky's bedroom—unlike her bedroom in our previous home—has no library at all, no books at all. She is alienated from that rich and welcoming world she contributed truth and elegance to. Becky could write a perfectly structured, flawlessly decorated, and marvelously coherent sentence that went on for seventy-five words—all without pomp, without verbosity, with grace, with truth, and which never overtaxed the reader's patience or intelligence. Now she never touches a keyboard or picks up a pen; she must fight a bloody war to secure the simplest word. She is muted. Words no longer serve her. Words fail her. She has been yanked away from the banquet of language and put on a starvation diet.

I have lost a literary companion and confidant. As I often told anyone who would listen, she made me a better writer, a better speaker, and a better person. I have not lost a child, but Rachel's lament is mine as well:

> This is what the LORD says:
> "A voice is heard in Ramah,
>   mourning and great weeping,

Rachel weeping for her children
                and refusing to be comforted,
                because they are no more." (Jeremiah 31:15)

I cannot imitate David's mourning for his infant son. I do not understand it. After Nathan had exposed his sins of adultery and murder, God caused the infant son conceived by David and Beer-sheba to die.

> Then David got up from the ground. After he had washed, put on lotions and changed his clothes, he went into the house of the Lord and worshiped. Then he went to his own house, and at his request they served him food, and he ate.
>
> His attendants asked him, "Why are you acting this way? While the child was alive, you fasted and wept, but now that the child is dead, you get up and eat!"
>
> He answered, "While the child was still alive, I fasted and wept. I thought, 'Who knows? The Lord may be gracious to me and let the child live.' But now that he is dead, why should I go on fasting? Can I bring him back again? I will go to him, but he will not return to me." (2 Samuel 12:20-23)

Sometimes, God may give release from grieving suddenly, although I know of no other such case either inside or outside of Scripture. David lost his son quickly. There is nothing quick about the decline demanded by dementia. Time slows down as misery speeds up. But I find a paradox. Every new setback seems to come raging in on the heels of the previous one—pain on pain, pain after pain—in this footrace to oblivion. But the footrace is a slow marathon, as my counselor keeps telling me: "Prepare for a marathon." Looking at Becky sometimes quickly transports me to better times—days of words and riposte—that don't seem so far away. But they are. We are stumbling through the long twilight, leading to night, but followed by light eternal. "There will be no more night. They will not need the light of a lamp or the light of the sun, for the Lord God will give them light. And they will reign for ever and ever" (Revelation 22:5).

On that day, every holy creature will worship the Word made flesh with all the fluency, intelligence, and feeling that is his due. Words will not fail us then, because the living Word, Christ Jesus, has never failed us. As the enraptured revelator, John, reported,

> After this I looked, and there before me was a great multitude that no one could count, from every nation, tribe, people and language, standing before the throne and before the Lamb. They were wearing white robes and were holding palm branches in their hands. And they cried out in a loud voice:
>
> > "Salvation belongs to our God,
> > who sits on the throne,
> > and to the Lamb."
>
> All the angels were standing around the throne and around the elders and the four living creatures. They fell down on their faces before the throne and worshiped God, saying:
>
> > "Amen!
> > Praise and glory
> > and wisdom and thanks and honor
> > and power and strength
> > be to our God for ever and ever.
> > Amen!" (Revelation 7:9-12)[2]

Eighteen

MY ESCAPE
INTO MEANING

I WANT TO ESCAPE my dementia-inflicted torments and find meaning elsewhere. But I cannot shirk responsibilities. Becky and I made vows before God Almighty in 1984. Our friends and family heard them. I must do my best to keep them. But I realized soon after Becky's diagnosis that I could not be her full-time caregiver. I had to work to make a living. I was too young to retire and not independently wealthy. (How many philosophers are?) Being a philosopher gives me satisfaction, direction, and meaning. I don't want to escape my job, since it is my calling. Let me explain and then move into other areas of life-sustaining and life-giving meaning.[1]

I cannot deny the meaning of my vocation, which remains strong and resilient. "Philosopher" is my title. To be a philosopher is God's calling on my life, and it is my career. My precocious young friend Liam asked me if I was a philosopher. "Yes," I replied. He continued, "What do philosophers do?" "We think a lot about arguments," I said. That seemed to satisfy him, and it satisfied me.

But philosophy is deeper than arguments, since it also summons reflection on the grisly vicissitudes of life, what breaks the heart and binds it back together. Philosophy originally was a discipline for finding out how to live, not just how to think well.

I am that rare person who has found my vocation and avocation to be one. I need not escape into trivial diversions to compensate for my day job. As Robert Frost put it in "Two Tramps in Mud Time" (1934):

> My object in living is to unite
> My avocation and my vocation
> As my two eyes make one in sight.
> Only where love and need are one,
> And the work is play for mortal stakes,
> Is the deed ever really done
> For Heaven and the future's sakes.

I do what I love, and it usually benefits others. There is no need to escape my job, since research and teaching and mentoring is where I flourish. The gifts given to me of teaching and writing have been confirmed, as Howard Hendricks would say, by finding people with the gifts of benefiting from my teaching and writing. I like to think that I am philosophical in all that I do, but I am not always writing about or teaching the discipline. I must attend to Becky, which, despite my love for her, is often exhausting and emotionally costly. I must sometimes escape. Only God can attend to all things at once. A Canadian philosopher helped me learn to attend rightly.

Media critic Marshall McLuhan did not celebrate the technological shifts he idiosyncratically analyzed for several decades. He was a phrasemaker—"the medium is the message" and "global village" are his—and a seer into the lineaments of the digital age. (He is listed on the masthead of *Wired* magazine as its "patron saint.") McLuhan was a conservative Roman Catholic and lamented most of the transformations he limned, particularly the rise of the image and the decline of the text. The media maven who became an academic celebrity (not many of those left) despaired of being able to stop or slow down these trends. His solace, besides his religion, was the "escape into understanding," which is the title of his authorized biography.[2]

For McLuhan, this aphoristic phrase (he spun out many) meant that by understanding complex social change, we find meaning rooted in understanding and, thus, escape its ruthless domination over the mind. Though he could not halt changes he discerned, he could find meaning in understanding them (at least in part). To use William Blake's phrase, "the mind-forg'd manacles" may fall away—even if one cannot fully break free from technology's atmosphere. One philosophical insight overcomes many existential failures. I have adjusted his language a bit by speaking of the *escape into meaning*, which, of course, involves understanding, but also activities.

I explained "the escape into meaning" to one of the students I mentor. It was a new insight for him (as it was for me about twenty years ago), which he related to many friends over the months. "I talk about that idea all the time with people," he told me. Yes, there is something to it, and it offers balm to roughed-up and wounded souls. It does to mine.

Escapism and *escapist* are not commendations. But in "a world of pain and fire and steel," we must escape.[3] Given the fall, escape is necessary. One cannot wade in the muck all the time. If kidnapped, one strives to escape. Tolkien said it best in "On Fairy Stories":

> Why should a man be scorned if, finding himself in prison, he tries to get out and go home? Or if, when he cannot do so, he thinks and talks about other topics than jailers and prison-walls?

The world outside has not become less real because the prisoner cannot see it. In using escape in this way the critics have chosen the wrong word, and, what is more, they are confusing, not always by sincere error, the Escape of the Prisoner with the Flight of the Deserter.[4]

I am not one for fairy stories and have felt dutifully guilty for at least thirty-five years for not reading *The Lord of the Rings*. In the daily crush of Becky's dementia, I live in the tension between "the Escape of the Prisoner" and "the Flight of the Deserter." I can flip back and forth like a twitchy toggle switch.

The deserter is easy to find and his modes of desertion are many. One may dive into addictions and obsessions—anything that shifts the mind from misery to nonmisery—it may not even be happiness. I don't have tight statistics, but divorce is often the escape for a spouse. Marriages afflicted by chronic illness often melt in the fires of despair, anger, and frustration. I have endured the feeling of "I cannot take it anymore" countless times—sometimes several times a day. Occasionally, it is more than a thought, but a scream. I scream less now than I did for the first few months after Becky's diagnosis. I am a teacher, after all, so I have to protect *my* voice, and my soul. And God is not hard of hearing. "Does he who fashioned the ear not hear? / Does he who formed the eye not see?" (Psalm 94:9).

Consider the escape into meaning. Since there is meaning aplenty, there are various forms of escape, if one can find them and open the gates. Most have a hobby of sorts, a discipline or activity reserved for leisure. However, there are immoral hobbies aplenty, such as collecting pornographic films or refining one's gambling talents. If a hobby does not hinder one's duties and refreshes the soul without hurting others, it is likely moral. Play is essential to work as long as we don't play at our work and work at our play. Riding a hobby too hard will wreck the hobby as a hobby; it may become an obsession and will injure the rider as well. When an aficionado becomes an addict, enjoyment is devoured by compulsion.

When I cannot reflect on or try to alleviate Becky's condition, I consider realms of meaning *outside of suffering*. Yes, I realize that there is meaning *within suffering*, and in my better moments I try to smelt meaning from suffering. The smelting may be slow-going and backbreaking work, burning the hands and filling the lungs with acrid smoke. But just as a person cannot exercise all the time, I need a respite, as do all caregivers. In fact, *respite care* is a crucial component in caring for a sick family member.

Given that I am an academic, I am sometimes asked what I read "for fun." This stumps me, since I enjoy most of what I read. Further, my life work of writing, teaching, and preaching is an oasis of significance at the center of my difficult life, and it all requires reading. My reading is integrated into my calling. Because of my many interests, I hope I am interesting without being overbearing or ostentatious. Howard Hendricks said that the best way to begin evangelistic discussions is simply to have wide interests that can interact with just about anyone else's interests.

My library is both a refuge and a rebuke to me. Long ago I switched from saying "my books" to "my library." Having a library, after all, is more dignified than merely having vast tracks of books. The question "Have you read all of them?" has been asked of me so often that I began to say, "No. But this is my library." Since no one has read every book in any public library, I am thus excused. The venerable Vernon Grounds had a library of many thousands of volumes, which is now incorporated into the Denver Seminary library. He was gifted with a photographic memory. When asked if he had read all his books, he replied, "No. But I want people to think that I have." I steal his line often. When asked if he has read all the books in his sprawling library, my professor friend Don Simpson replies, "I have read some of them twice." I will remember that line.

My interests are almost encyclopedic, so much of the world beckons from my library: philosophy, theology, religious studies, psychology, history, art, jazz, biography, dogs, literature, sociology, poetry, books on grammar and style, and more. I am an intellectual omnivore. My books—let alone my journals, magazines, and newspapers—are my friends, even if the unread ones taunt me and beg for my attention. As I get older, I give away more unread books, knowing I will never get to them.

Books have unique charms that cannot be replaced by digitized information. Most books bear meaning graciously. Books can be held. They have a history in time and space as physical objects. Each page has but one set of inscriptions, unlike screens, which can present an unlimited number. This insures heft.[5] In 1976 I read a book that influenced my ministry: *The God Who Is There* by Francis Schaeffer. That very book is in my library forty years later. It is an integral aspect of my life, and I reread it often because it anchors me in a meaning and vision that is stronger than my sorrows over Becky.

I read about nearly everything, but I also use my eyes to behold several forms of nontextual art, principally twentieth-century painting, even at its strangest and most perplexing. I had touched this world before, mostly through the writings of Francis Schaeffer and Hans Rookmaaker. But I did not embrace it, as I began to do several years ago. Becky was yet to be diagnosed as having dementia, but the early signs—along with all her other ills—were there and worsening. So, I escaped into new and intriguing meanings.

For the thoughtful person, the escape makes its kind and challenging demands. For me to appreciate painting, for example, I must *receive* it before I evaluate it or even enjoy it fully. That is, I try to take it for what it is on its own terms, eschewing any cheap *use* of the painting for my diversion, delight, or entertainment. I learned this distinction from a neglected work by C. S. Lewis, *An Experiment in Criticism*. Lewis contrasted those who read to pass the time with those who love literature (fiction and nonfiction), who chart their lives by its revelations. When experiencing any form of art worth experiencing, I want to receive it, to let it do its work on me. This can be the gateway to the profound, to dimensions hitherto unknown and unsavored.

An essay by Marva Dawn has assisted my escape into meaning also. In the short essay "Behold," she considers the mode of attention in which we do not merely *see* or *hear* or *touch*.[6] Rather, we apprehend something with reverence and respect (if it is so worthy). Consider John the Baptizer, who testified to Christ in good King James English, "Behold the Lamb of God, which taketh away the sin of the world" (John 1:29 KJV). We should not merely see or be in the presence of the Lamb of God, but rather *behold* him. Twentieth-century art, in general, is far from Christocentric, but I gave it a chance by trying to behold it.

My sense of twentieth-century art before had been generally negative. Modernism in art was nihilistic, destroying previous forms and traditions. Indeed, it often did. John Cage, for example, often attempted to create music by chance and arranged sounds in something other than music, classically construed.[7] Perhaps he was more a jester than a composer. I have not warmed to him, but I now explore the meanings of abstract expressionism (for example, Jackson Pollack and Lee Krasner), cubism (early Picasso), and color field painting (Mark Rothko), all of which is endlessly engrossing and fills the senses in new, uncharted, and unexplored ways.

Becky was never attracted by any aspect of aesthetic modernism.[8] When the classical radio station played almost any twentieth-century music, she would mock it (making a few dissonant sounds) before promptly turning it off. I did this too. We also scorned nontraditional forms of painting as "weird," although we knew little about it. (Uninformed ridicule can be great fun—as can informed ridicule.)

One day Becky looked through one of my many books on modern nonrepresentational painting and was fascinated. She now sometimes visits the Denver Art Museum when her brother John or best friend Sharon visits. Her tastes—however attenuated by dementia—have broadened a bit even as her once-luminous intellect lessens.

While Becky does not study modern painting, I do. As a philosopher, I explore the meaning of paintings in relation to the painter's worldview and their philosophy of art. As T. S. Eliot urged, I pursue an "educated taste." I can be lost in these works without fear of falling into a pit or meeting predators.

Out of many cases, consider the paintings of Mark Rothko, who, later in his career, invented a new form of painting, sometimes referred to as the "color field" (although Rothko did not appreciate that moniker). These works, often large, consist of rectangles placed on each other, situated in a subtly glowing ambience. Words fail a bit. Please look for yourself by viewing them online, in a book, or, best yet, at an exhibit. Here, we can stand or sit before a Rothko and let it sink into pores previously unknown. But please don't rush by. You are not in an automobile.

Another painter ministers directly and deeply to those feeling the heavy weight of the fall. A few years ago, while illustrating a concept with several of his works, I told my students that Georges Rouault had "saved my life," especially in 2012 and 2013. Rouault, like Rothko, imagined a unique and compelling style, reminiscent of stained-glass figures. Unlike Rothko, Rouault was drawn to human figures, especially faces, which he drew with large, impasto strokes. His genius lay in depicting tragedy kindly. While Picasso (perhaps a nihilist) represented the fragmentation of the twentieth century with odd images of discombobulated bodies, Rouault looked at the tragic side of life with compassion. He painted prostitutes, ugly judges, old kings, and sad clowns in his inimitable style. It is not surprising that Rouault was a Christian. Like Blaise Pascal before him, he painted both the majesty and misery of humanity, but, at least until his later work, focused on the darkness that enshrouds God's good world. Through Rouault, I can escape into the deepest meaning of all: the gospel. I thank God for opening this door to me in my distress.

Outside of reading and painting, music (live and recorded) is my chief escape into meaning. It is for Becky also, but not in the same way. Although I may bang on a drum set, I am not a musician, nor do I know much about musical theory. Becky was a singer and a pianist. She could read music. When Becky sings old gospel songs with her music therapist or her caregiver, she is transported: her face changes and the words come naturally. When I cannot think of anything else to help her cope, I put on a classical or religious recording.

My romance with music is both affective and cognitive. Since music expresses and encourages emotion and sparks thought, it frames our consciousness with aural meaning. It transports us to other dwellings. The best music has a transcendent quality; it is other and better that what we typically experience. This is why we may close our eyes while listening: we want our sensations to narrow to that sound. No wonder, since God was there when "the morning stars sang together / and all the angels shouted for joy" (Job 38:7). In music, we join a heavenly chorus, either in concord or discord. Neurological descriptions of our brain states while listening to music cannot rob us of that irreducible, first-person experience of that which is beyond the first-person.

Beholding musicians making music adds another dimension to the escape into meaning. I will speak only of jazz, since I am an initiate and aficionado. Finding the essence of jazz is vexing, but its essence involves improvisation.[9] In small combos, each musician solos, but the entire group is improvising. In jazz, there is no *backup band*. I attended a concert of the Larry Golding's Trio at Dazzle, my favorite jazz club in Denver. During a solo, guitarist Peter Bernstein played a phase that Bill Steward, while keeping the beat, mimicked on drums. They did not even acknowledge each other with a nod or a wink, but they conversed through the notes. I hear it and smile. There were many smiles that night. It gets better when I bring a student or friend who is new to jazz or a novice. Then I can teach as well as behold. One jazz epiphany delivered a pure and radiant joy that left dementia and all its ills far, far behind.

I took a young couple to Dazzle to hear the Cyrus Chestnut Trio. We savored every minute, but a few minutes stood out. Chestnut, playing the piano with his back to the drummer, finished a solo, turned around, looked at his young drummer, and started scat singing! He scatted and stopped. The drummer answered. It was call and response, another indelible feature of real jazz. I turned to my young jazz neophytes, laughed, and rubbed the top of Michael's head, who was laughing along with his wife. This odd musical exchange—I had never heard this paring of scat and drums before—was made sweeter because young, newlywed Cassie is a *sibling in suffering*. By this, I mean she's a soul who has suffered in extraordinary ways, ways that most cannot imagine. Her family member suffers from a rare and horrible disease that keeps him from a productive life and, at unpredictable times, physically endangers those around him. But dear Cassie was laughing with her husband and with me as we joined the fellowship of jazz. Moments like these do nothing to take away the suffering I will return to, but they are glad antidotes for agonies.

No one can exhaust the topic of music—its forms, history, relation to other aspects of culture, and theological meaning. I agree with Duke Ellington that there are only two kinds of music: good music and the other kind. I am puzzled by a friend who seldom listens to music and has never developed his taste for music. Puzzling though it is, I know this godly man escapes into meaning as well. He simply visits other regions of that vast land. And he and I and Becky know that one day we will not just *visit* this foreign land. We will call it home. When there, we will need no escape from the veil of tears, since we will dwell there forever, enjoying music and every good sensory enjoyment, and "the wealth of the nations" will be brought in.[10]

> Your gates will always stand open,
>> they will never be shut, day or night,
> so that people may bring you the wealth of the nations—
>> their kings led in triumphal procession. (Isaiah 60:11)

The apogee and acme of all enjoyment will be God himself, the greatest Composer, Arranger, and Performer of all. His supremacy will become our felicity forever.

Since so many caregivers suffer burnout and take rotten refuge in that which is forbidden by God, I offer my escapes into meaning perhaps not so much as examples of *what to do* but, rather, as *ways to be*. Atheists to the contrary, this broken world has meaning: activities worth doing, thoughts worth thinking, feelings worth having, and culture worth appreciating—by oneself or with others. God is the giver of all good gifts, even gifts of *escape*. But *defections* from the love of God and neighbor are not among them.

Interlude

BECKY AS MY STUDENT

BECKY WAS QUITE INVOLVED at Denver Seminary for about the first ten years of my time as a professor. She gave lectures in several courses and was a student in several of my offerings. She was not an average student, but the smartest person (professor included) in the room. And she felt no deference toward the professor. Becky was a stickler for intellectual precision and could abide no fog in the room, however confidently I may have spewed it. Becky kept me intellectually accountable (with humor) in ways that no one else could. (It was the same when she edited my writing.) Twenty years later, one of my students harks back to this with glee nearly every time I see him. Yes, those were salad days of intellect and repartee for both of us.

However, as Becky's general health declined, she kept more to herself and seldom attended any of my courses, sermons, or public lectures. She was my best critic—utterly honest, discerning, and kind. After I had given a message at a prestigious evangelical church a few years before Becky's diagnosis, I was eager for Becky to see it online. After watching it intently, she simply said to me, "It was astonishingly articulate." There was no higher human praise for me. (She didn't notice that I made a reference to "Chronicles 12:32," without saying if it was First or Second Chronicles.)[1]

Recently, Becky attended my class at Denver Seminary on the philosophy of Blaise Pascal. She was acquainted with this French genius through my many writings about him. Our friend Naomi took her there.

This is heartening and distressing. Becky has trouble occupying herself. Things she did, she cannot do, since her faculties are limited. Dementia has made her illiterate. Thus, getting out of the house to be with Naomi and hear me teach is good for her. She has told me she enjoys it. This is heartening, especially since I sometimes feel I am not doing enough to help her be more active.

Seeing Becky in my class is distressing. She does not seem uncomfortable; she does not look tired; she sometimes looks at me with a dim twinkle in her eye. I may mention something she has said or written pertinent to the class discussion. Even if she does not remember, it is fine, since the students know of and share in (to some extent) our grief, and because Becky is used to forgetting. It does not embarrass her. I know that Becky listens, but she cannot understand and critique as she did even a few years ago. Her face has changed. Her wide range of sharp expressions has softened into a dull but grateful look of acceptance. She still laughs—and at the right times—but the laugh does not sparkle with intelligence, and it is not followed by a hilarious comment of her own.

I first came to know Becky when she was my student at the University of Oregon when we were both in campus ministry. Soon I realized she was my intellectual equal; not long after that she was my intellectual superior. For a long time after, she was an integral part of my intellectual development and ministry as my editor and adviser. Now Becky has become my student again. After one of my lectures, Becky and I had a late dinner at home. She said, "You are really smart." I replied, "I have to be. It's my job." We both laughed.

Now I need not fear her penetrating questions and cannot hope for her astute observations. She is there, but she is not there. I am there with her, but I am not there with her in the same way I was with her when she was my best student, my intellectual duelist, and the wry and dry wit who had the inside scoop on the professor.

Nineteen

HOW IS BECKY?

I sometimes get lost walking through dementia's twilight. The trail may be torturous and the walking is often more like staggering. But I soldier on, marching while wounded, heaving for good air. But Becky and I need other soldiers to hold us up and to call us on. Every sufferer needs the same. What might you do to show compassion to those trudging down suffering's road? Or how might we accidentally add weight to their burden?

"How is Becky?" I have heard this hundreds of times. Even before dementia, Becky has been chronically ill for decades. Most people I know are concerned and want to show their concerns. It often fails. When someone says, "Is Becky better?" this demands a difficult response. Since I am honest to a fault, I say no, and give a reluctant and uncomfortable explanation. Recently, someone who knows the downward road my wife is on asked, "Is Becky better?" I wearily answered, "No. She is not going to get better, but we are hanging on." We were embarrassed. Perhaps those who ask this want to offer some optimism to those mired in misery. But mere optimism without intelligent sympathy only rubs the wound rawer. I feel that I should give an excuse for why a loved one is not getting better. Confessing the truth also lets the questioner down, so I feel responsible for depressing someone.

I like it better when people simply ask how we are doing and then leave time for an honest answer. I remember my aged grandfather being asked how he was doing. He would often say, "Terrible," then laugh. The laugh did not annul the answer. For me, "hanging in there," "surviving," "I've been worse" are my answers for people I know. Or I may simply say, "Please pray for us." Occasionally, I say, "Very good," and mean it. While I was staying at the Rochester, Minnesota, L'Abri for rest and teaching, I said this to a young friend over the phone, who was shocked and delighted to hear it. She knew I meant it. My most theological answer is, "I am hanging by a thread, but the thread is knit by God." This often surprises people, since it is so long and theological. So be it. I don't like clichés.

My wife has been so sick for so long that "How's Becky?" has become oppressive to me, because she is never doing well. At times, it is more compassionate to ask nothing and simply greet someone, touch them appropriately, or assure them that you are praying for them (if you are). A friend of mine suffers terribly on account of her sibling's extreme foolishness, which endangers her child and exasperates the sister's parents. I no longer ask about this, since I know the subject is awful. I say nothing, but wait for a report.

Americans are characteristically entrepreneurial and optimistic. This is a strength and a weakness. "Never give in—never, never, never, never!" we say with Churchill. But if we are too optimistic, we give the wounded soul no time to grieve. We want to cheer people up and help them (as is so often said) *move forward*. Americans always want to *move forward*, even if it is not the right direction to move. Moving forward at the end of a cliff is not advisable. Cheerful people are usually skilled at cheering up others, but cheerfulness can backfire. Two good friends of mine are consistently cheerful, as was the late philosopher Gordon Lewis, a friend and colleague. But none of them would bypass sympathy to rush toward levity or frivolity. They realize that they cannot tickle anyone into happiness when the person is contorted by pain. Nor should we shove people past grief and into diversions or evasions.

On April 20, 1999, at Columbine High School in Littleton, Colorado, two teenagers murdered thirteen people and wounded more than twenty others before fatally shooting themselves. This was, at the time, the deadliest school shooting in American history. The popular novelist Danielle Steel wrote an editorial for the *Rocky Mountain News*, offering solace to the grieving.[1] After her young son's suicide in 1997, she was told that she should get over it because it had been *six weeks* since he died. It once took me six weeks to fully recover from a contusion on my right leg. No bona fide human being can recover from their child's suicide in six weeks. Steele counseled that we should let grief take its unpredictable course and not rush to admonishment. She writes, "We still miss him. Enormously. You don't stop missing someone you lose, but you learn to live with it, like a limb you lose."[2]

I told someone that Becky has dementia. He was saddened and surprised. But he quickly said that it might not be that bad. His father had Alzheimer's and became obliviously happy near the end. I told him that Alzheimer's affects the brain differently than primary progressive aphasia. (How I hate that phrase of doom.) We did not anticipate a happy oblivion. He gave cold comfort, but from a warm heart, I am sure. It did not help, but I am sure his subsequent prayers did.

Perhaps the bitterest way to disappoint a person trying to navigate through twilight is to offer help, but not give it. In their concern to aid, some make empty promises. We live within the grasp of promises kept and suffer when they are broken. This may be a minor annoyance or a heart-rending disappointment. Immanuel Kant argued that breaking a promise is uniformly wrong. I take this to be a mistake in the right direction. Most promises should be honored. The psalmist commends the person who keeps a good promise, who "honoureth them that fear the LORD. He that sweareth to his own hurt, and changeth not" (Psalm 15:4 KJV). We have promises to keep. The Preacher knew this: "It is better not to make a vow than to make one and not fulfill it" (Ecclesiastes 5:5).

However, we should break promises made in haste or on the basis of false information. Martin Luther promised, even vowed, to commit his entire life to a Catholic monastery. But because of his glad discovery of the gospel, God called him to be a great reformer.

Some take themselves to be heroes of helping, and promise what they cannot fulfill. I know from sad experience. If someone comes to their moral senses and asks for forgiveness, we should grant it, even with a broken heart. It seems that few—myself included—know quite what to do with the unusual and irksome imperatives of dementia. We are lost, treading on alien ground that threatens to crack open and suck us down, as in a violent earthquake. But being lost together, bound by wise promises, keeps us from plummeting out of sight. We are lost in God's world, but have not lost the race. God has not lost us.

I may feel lost. But I am not a lost soul. Neither is Becky. I wish Becky were here in the way she was before this slow-motion anguish began for both of us. I once insisted to Becky in a stressful situation, "I am lost without you." Not long after, I began to slowly lose Becky. I am losing her, but I am not lost. In the final analysis, she is not lost either. Jesus pronounced, "The Son of Man came to seek and to save the lost" (Luke 19:10). Since he sought and saved us long ago, we will not be lost to his love or power. Still, it hurts to lose so much of what I knew of Becky. And I need others to help me find my bearings and weep with me.

Wounded, Risen One
by Rebecca Merrill Groothuis

Your body
    stretched and wretched
  draped upon the instrument of your death.

Your soul
    plummeting precipitously,
        spinning
    in the dizzying darkness.

A hell you'd never known, and
        could not have imagined;
The claustrophobic horror
      of the howling black night,
    the consuming stench of death;
The deep narrow light-less place
           of sin
      that is not your own.

You never knew it could be like this;
    you can hardly breathe.
You feel your heart tear open,
    a deep, jagged break through the center.
"Oh no, oh God, my *God*,
    why have you forsaken me?"

But God
    did not abandon you
    in the pit, the pain,
      of a sin not your own.

Miraculously
   your soul returned to the light
      (though death had been so utterly complete);
   your wretchedness
            moved behind you;
      night gave way to dawn.

Life resurrected.

As the fresh, clean scent of morning
      fills your lungs,
   you wonder—had you,
               just the other night,
      been breathing the stale filth
         of hell's depths?

Your fingers reach for
      your side, your palms.
In your soul you feel
   the long scar
      where the wound had gaped
               and bled
      but now was clean and closed.

Knowing the past
      you leave the past
and press ahead to the new thing
      that your God, my God,
         is doing:
   cleaning and closing
      the wounds of our separation

from your holiness,
drawing us into purity
and maturity
—resurrection life!

Yet you remember
—you will always remember—
the dark night of your wounding.
For it changes everything.

And through the haze of its pain
a new light now shines.

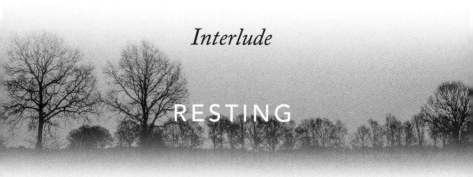

Interlude

RESTING

FOR MANY YEARS BECKY AND I would rest together. She would lie on her back and I would put my head on her chest. Normally we would not fall asleep, but simply enjoy each other's company. As Becky's distress over her dementia has increased, these peaceful times have decreased. But Becky has little to do now. So, one night I went up to her bedroom and said we should relax as we used to. She liked the idea, but had difficulty knowing how to move over into an appropriate spot on the bed. I helped her, and we were back in that old *no-worry-just-relax zone*, enjoying each other's closeness.

I would discuss a few things and Becky would respond simply, sometimes by laughing. Sunny had been realizing lately that Becky was more unhappy and less able to fend for herself. When he came upstairs, he jumped up on the bed and licked us, tail wagging, but not from happiness. After nuzzling us, he lay down at the foot of the bed with his head resting on my foot. We were all just *being* and not trying to fix anything. We could *do* this merely by *being*.

After several minutes, I looked into Becky's eyes. I saw an innocence, peace, and love that I had not seen in years. Everything else dropped off—no questions, no worries, no fears. There was love, our love revealed in a look I had not seen during the years when debility devoured simple pleasures and painted a pained narrative over every good thing.

That look of love warmed me, still warms me as I write. For now, love was not squashed, pummeled, chopped to bloody bits by circumstance. I breathed it in during just a moment, and began to weep. But this weeping did not stem from anger or fear. I did not feel that. These tears were sweet. They did not burn. They reconnected me with our love for each other that was overgrown by the detritus of the fall. In that moment, all of our pure enjoyment over the years came back, and I realized it would never return.

Becky asked me why I was crying. "Tell me what's wrong," she kindly said. "It is everything," I replied. "Everything" was a common cause for lament and crying for years. Why mention each good thing taken away and each bad thing added? "Everything" covered it. To this she laughed an odd but apt laugh. She understands the depths of this word for us.

For about an hour after seeing her pure face of love, I wept every time her image came back into my mind. There was a sweet suffering in these tears.

Conclusion

FROM TWILIGHT
INTO DARKNESS

WE HAVE WALKED MANY MILES through twilight in these pages. I have walked more miles than I have recounted, miles of silence and regret. The road will become steeper, rockier, and less word-filled. I don't expect to write about what's next—when I leave the twilight and enter thick darkness. Dawn and day follow night. But that night is long.

The twilight has been long for Becky and me. My last lament is that I have not done enough. I have not been enough. The voices say, "You should have spent more time with Becky. You should have pursued more doctors. You should have done more to keep Becky busy. You should have never raised your voice. You should not have depended so heavily on that friend. You should have . . . You should not have . . ."

But another voice says, "Yes and no." I can neither find nor write a roadmap for this death march into ever-deeper lament. My checklists are written in anguished ink. I cannot keep up. I am not a relativist, but there is no one right way to live through this. Each person with dementia is different, physically and psychologically; each caregiver is different; every situation is different. There is no roadmap, but there are detours to avoid: anger, selfishness, self-pity, rage, cowardice, dissipation, laziness, and the worst detour of all—deserting your post.

But "love is as strong as death" (Song of Songs 8:6), and stronger. We know this because of an innocent man nailed to a Roman pike of shame, festooned by a dying criminal on each side. That young man died and was buried. Three days later, his tomb was emptied of death and he was found more alive than any of us are right now. These matchless and unmatchable events—written in books, but resident in reality—are my only hope in life and death, in Becky's life and in Becky's death. Jesus is Lord.

As I dare to look ahead—and I must, if I am not to desert my post—I cannot consult a road map; I cannot turn on a GPS, but I can find fuel in love. Because of Christ, Paul's discourse is not in vain; it is not mere romanticism. It is backed by a reality we do not see, but is nevertheless incandescent and undying.

> If I speak in the tongues of men and of angels, but have not love, I am a noisy gong or a clanging cymbal. And if I have prophetic powers, and understand all mysteries and all knowledge, and if I have all faith, so as to remove mountains, but have not love, I am nothing. If I give away all I have, and if I deliver my body to be burned, but have not love, I gain nothing.
>
> Love is patient and kind; love is not jealous or boastful; it is not arrogant or rude. Love does not insist on its own way; it is not irritable or resentful; it does not rejoice at wrong, but rejoices in the right. Love bears all things, believes all things, hopes all things, endures all things.

Love never ends; as for prophecies, they will pass away; as for tongues, they will cease; as for knowledge, it will pass away. For our knowledge is imperfect and our prophecy is imperfect; but when the perfect comes, the imperfect will pass away. When I was a child, I spoke like a child, I thought like a child, I reasoned like a child; when I became a man, I gave up childish ways. For now we see in a mirror dimly, but then face to face. Now I know in part; then I shall understand fully, even as I have been fully understood. So faith, hope, love abide, these three; but the greatest of these is love. (1 Corinthians 13 RSV)

ACKNOWLEDGMENTS

I AM INDEBTED TO CINDY BUNCH, who gently and wisely helped me craft a bulky manuscript into a memoir.

I extend thanks to the many souls who pray for Rebecca and me and who prayed for the writing of his book.

Most of all, I acknowledge the intelligence, wit, wisdom, and faith of my wife, Rebecca Merrill Groothuis, who lives day by day through the unthinkable.

Appendix

LIGHTENING THE LOAD

Humans living this side of the fall and before heaven are quite skilled at making situations worse. I will not count all the ways but instead speak of what has helped Becky and me, and what may lighten the load a bit for others.[1]

There is a time to simply sit with others in their grief, as Job's friends did at the beginning of his trials. Silence may not heal, but it does reduce the pains inflicted by a loose tongue. When life is beyond human repair, we should not try to repair it. Why trouble the air with futility? Why set up more lost hopes? Perhaps we need to suffer well with others instead of dispensing well-meaning but heartbreaking panaceas. How might we do this?

First, we ought to pray for wisdom before speaking or communicating with someone under the pressures of loss. Ask "the God of all comfort" to give you the heart and tongue that heals (or at least does not multiply the pain). Good intentions, though, may produce bad results. You do not say, "Are you grieving well?" to someone who just lost a spouse. We should grieve with the sorrowful heart, not ask it for an internal spiritual audit. Someone is diagnosed with cancer and is trying to reorient their life to handle it. But someone from their church says, "Oh, if I had to have chemotherapy—just shoot me." The person who received this body blow, nevertheless, prepared for chemotherapy with courage and hope. We should remember what the book of James says about the power of the tongue to make everything worse (James 3:1-12).

Second, we should avoid overinterpreting the dire situations of a fallen world by trying to read God's mind. This makes for hollow comfort. Yes, God will bring good out of evil for his people (Romans 8:28), but we don't quite know how he will do this. The silver lining of a dark cloud—if we can even find it—does not explain the full meaning of the suffering.

In light of this, we must learn to silently sit with our ignorance instead of spewing forth our pious pronouncements on the specifics of divine providence. Job's friends went wrong only when they broke their silence in his presence and began to speak without knowledge.

Third, learn to lament with people. I addressed lament throughout this book, but consider two points. Listen to the stories of the suffering and identify with them. Say unprofound but appropriate things like, "I am so sorry" and "That is terrible." It is not wise to try to cheer before it's time.

> Like one who takes away a garment on a cold day,
>> or like vinegar poured on a wound,
>> is one who sings songs to a heavy heart. (Proverbs 25:20)

The American South has an expression that captures this perfectly: "I hate it for you." I hate it that marriages are being ripped apart. I hate it that my friend's spouse is going through chemotherapy. I hate it for all of them, and I should show them that I hate it. I hate it because I love them. I especially hate it for Becky.

In most cases, it is not wise to say to the suffering one, "I know how you feel." This is because you probably do not. Proverbs guides us: "Each heart knows its own bitterness, / and no one else can share its joy" (Proverbs 14:10).

I know my own dementia-shaped bitterness. I know nothing of the wounded hearts of those who lose children to disease or disaster. People often say to me, "I have no idea how you feel." I appreciate that.

It is unwise to tell people that losing a spouse or having cancer or facing a divorce isn't really so bad. It is bad, very bad. This is a fallen world, a world that is still groaning in anticipation of its final redemption (Romans 8:18-26). As Nicholas Wolterstorff writes in his moving and profound meditation, *Lament for a Son*, we must sit on the mourner's bench with the suffering and lament with them. This in itself provides a kind of comfort.[2]

A delightfully antiquated and marvelous way to offer love to the sufferers is to write cards and letters of condolence. As I read cards, Facebook posts, and emails of condolence, I wonder what, exactly, makes for a kind condolence. A few elements come to mind. A condolence letter may address a death or a major loss of any kind, even the death of a pet. Christopher Hitchens, in his memoir, urges us not to postpone concern for others: "I can perhaps offer a crumb of counsel. If there is anybody known to you who might benefit from a letter or a visit, do not on any account postpone the writing or the making of it. The difference made will almost certainly be more than you have calculated."[3]

Genuine sorrow may not be captured by a prefabricated card. But if an appropriate greeting card is found (which is unlikely), it is best to add a few words in your own handwriting. Miss Manners, the maven of all things polite and impolite, disagrees, however: "Sympathy cards of any kind are in bad taste. Rotten taste. Only personal messages (a.k.a. real letters) are acceptable for concern such a personal sentiment as sympathy with the bereaved."[4] Your sorrow should not be despairing (which is the sin of giving up on God), but respectful and tender. However, it is never right to try to hurry one along to joy when they are still marinating in sorrow.

Another aspect of condolence is remembering and appreciating the life now over or in distress: a few words about the person's smile or laugh or kindness. This sparks bright memories that dispel a bit of the harsh darkness of death.

The better condolences also offer hope for the bereft, the bereaved, and the grieving; they offer some noncliché reason to believe your sorrow will lighten, your life will move into brighter places, that this death or devastation will one day be swallowed up in victory (if that can be said of the newly dead).

Other condolences are less wise; their vices include overused phrases robbed of meaning through overuse: "Earth's loss is heaven's gain," and so on. These are true, but trite. Better to use your own faltering words than to steal such stock phrases. Yes, it's the thought that counts, but why not try to match the right words with such sentiments?

Perhaps the most grievous failure in words of condolence is silence—no words at all. Those close to you and your beloved deceased write nothing. Why is this? Perhaps these souls are overwhelmed by the prospect of writing such weighty words. Instead of failing in this tough task, they succeed by doing nothing, claiming an inability that renders them mute. But this makes the bereaved even lonelier in their losses.

I am but a babe in this loving skill, suffering well with others. Will you join me in the school of lament? Will you learn to sit on the mourner's bench before God and with those whom you love?

RECOMMENDED READING ON LAMENT AND GRIEF

Card, Michael. *A Sacred Sorrow: Reaching Out to God in the Lost Language of Lament*. Colorado Springs: NavPress, 2005. Winsomely explains the biblical concept of lament.

Keller, Timothy. *Walking with God Through Pain and Suffering*. New York: Penguin Books, 2015. Argues that Christianity, of all the religions and philosophies, finds the most meaning in human suffering. Also gives sound advice on the practice of suffering well as a Christian.

Lewis, C. S. *A Grief Observed*. New York: HarperOne, 2001. An often agonizing but faith-affirming reflection on the loss of his wife from cancer.

Meyers, Jeffrey. *A Table in the Mist: Ecclesiastes Through New Eyes*. Monroe, LA: Athanasius Press, 2006. An able exposition and application of the biblical book that has helped me the most in my own lamentations.

Payne, Don J. *Surviving the Unthinkable: Choosing to Live After Someone You Love Chooses to Die*. Eugene, OR: Resource Publications, 2015. A short, moving, wise, and well-written account—with application behind coping with suicide.

Wolterstorff, Nicholas. *Lament for a Son*. Grand Rapids: Eerdmans, 1987. Wise reflections on the sudden death of Wolterstorff's son, who died in a mountain-climbing accident at the age twenty-five.

NOTES

INTRODUCTION

[1]Bertrand Russell, *Essays on Skepticism* (New York: Philosophical Press, 1962), 87.

[2]W. H. Auden, "Musée des Beaux Arts," in David Lehman, "Art's Lessons, Drawn in Verse," *Wall Street Journal*, May 14, 2016, C12.

CHAPTER 1: RAGE IN A PSYCH WARD

[1]Michel De Montaigne, "How the Soul Discharges its Emotions Against False Objects When Lacking Real Ones," *The Complete Essays*, trans. and ed. M. A. Screech (New York: Penguin, 2003), 19-21.

[2]Viktor Frankl, *Man's Search for Meaning*, rev. and updated (New York: Pocket Books, 1997), 135.

[3]Ibid., 86.

CHAPTER 6: THE TEMPTATION TO HATE GOD

[1]Bernard Schweizer, *Hating God: The Untold Story of Misotheism* (Oxford University Press, 2011), 8.

[2]Fyodor Dostoevsky, *The Karamazov Brothers*, trans. Ignat Avsey (New York: Oxford University Press, 1994), 298-99. Most translations use the title *The Brothers Karamazov*.

[3]Ibid., 308.

[4]C. S. Lewis, *A Grief Observed* (New York: Bantam Books, 1976), 4-5.

[5]See Douglas Groothuis, "The Moral Argument for God," *Christian Apologetics* (Downers Grove, IL: IVP Academic, 2011).

[6]Lewis, *Grief Observed*, 45-46.

[7]See Eugene Peterson, *Tell It Slant* (Grand Rapids: Eerdmans).

[8]This is also one of the central teachings of the book of Ecclesiastes. See Jeffrey Meyers, *A Table in the Mist: Ecclesiastes Through New Eyes* (Monroe, LA: Athanasius Press, 2006).

[9]William Backus, *The Hidden Rift with God* (Minneapolis: Bethany Book House, 1990).

CHAPTER 7: LEARNING TO LAMENT

[1]Blaise Pascal, *Pensées* 148, ed. Alban Krailsheimer (New York: Penguin, 1995), 74.

[2]The material in this chapter is adapted from Douglas Groothuis, "Learning to Lament," *Journal for Baptist Theology & Ministry* 10, no. 2 (fall 2013), 70-73.

[3]Blaise Pascal, "Prayer to Ask of God the Proper Use of Suffering," *Bartleby .com*, accessed March 15, 2017, www.bartleby.com/48/3/2.html.

[4]Martin Seligman, *Authentic Happiness* (New York: Atria Books, 2004).

[5]C. S. Lewis, *The Abolition of Man* (New York: Macmillan, 1976), 25.

[6]Todd Rungren, "Sometimes I Don't Know What to Feel," *A Wizard, a True Star*, 1973.

[7]Nicholas Wolterstorff, *Lament for a Son* (Grand Rapids: Eerdmans, 1987), 85.

[8]See Glen Pemberton, *Hurting With God* (Abilene, TX: Abilene Christian University Press, 2012).

[9]Eric Clapton, "Nobody Knows You When You're Down and Out," *Unplugged*, 1992.

[10]John Van Sloten, *The Day Metallica Came to Church: Searching for the Everywhere God in Everything* (Grand Rapids: Square Inch Press, 2010).

[11]C. S. Lewis, *The Screwtape Letters* (San Francisco: HarperSanFrancisco, 2001), 40.

[12]John Piper has written many books on this theme. See especially his *Desiring God: Meditations of a Christian Hedonist*, rev. ed. (Colorado Springs: Multnomah Press, 2011). Piper's *When I Don't Desire God* (Wheaton, IL: Crossway, 2013) is helpful for those mired in lament.

CHAPTER 8: JOY IN LAMENT

[1]Stuart C. Smith, *Dead to Sin, Alive to God: Discover the Power of Reckoning to Set You Free in Christ* (Eugene, OR: Resource Publications, 2016).

CHAPTER 9: MOSES AND OUR SADNESS

[1]Blaise Pascal, *Pensées*, ed. Alban Krailsheimer (New York: Penguin, 1995), 165.

[2]Atul Gawande, *Being Mortal: Medicine and What Matters in the End* (New York: Metropolitan Books, 2014).

[3]Christopher Hitchens, *Mortality* (New York: Twelve, 2012).

[4]John Newton, "Amazing Grace," 1779.

CHAPTER 13: LEARNING TO LIE TO MY WIFE (AS LITTLE AS POSSIBLE)

[1]C. S. Lewis, *The Screwtape Letters* (New York: Macmillan, 1961), 26-27.

[2]Augustine, "Lying," in Harry G. Frankfort, *On Bullsh*t* (Princeton, NJ: Princeton University Press, 2005), 58.

CHAPTER 14: GALLOWS HUMOR

[1]Monty Python, "Miss Ann Elk," *Monty Python's Previous Record*, 1972.

[2]I am drawing from D. H. Monro, "Humor," *The Encyclopedia of Philosophy*, ed. Paul Edwards (New York: MacMillan, 1967), 4:90-93.

[3]Wayne F. Hill and Cynthia J. Ottchen, *Shakespeare's Insults: Educating Your Wit* (New York: Crown Trade Paperbacks, 1991), 116.

[4]*The Pink Panther Strikes Again*, 1976.

[5]See A. W. Tozer, "The Use and Abuse of Humor," *Of God and Men* (Chicago: Moody Publishers, 2015).

[6]"Gallows Humour," *Oxford Living Dictionaries*, accessed March 16, 2017, https://en.oxforddictionaries.com/definition/gallows_humour.

[7]See Irving Goffman, "Total Institutions," in *Asylums: Essays on the Social Situation of Mental Patients and Other Inmates* (New York: Anchor Books, 1961). These large institutions were disbanded in the 1960s, but the defining features of a "total institution" remain in many instances. See E. Fuller Torrey, *The Insanity Offense: How America's Failure to Treat the Seriously Mentally Ill Endangers Its Citizens* (New York: W. W. Norton, 2012).

CHAPTER 15: DOGS, DEMENTIA, AND US

[1]See also 2 Kings 8:13; Exodus 22:31; 2 Samuel 3:8; Proverbs 26:11; 2 Samuel 9:8.

[2]James Thurber, *Thurber's Dogs* (New York: Simon & Schuster, 1955), 205.

[3]Roger Scruton spends the chapter "Life with Sam" of his autobiography on his dog, Sam. See his *Gentle Regrets* (New York: Bloomsbury Academic, 2006).

[4]See Alexandra Horowitz, "Belonging to the Home," *Inside of a Dog: What Dogs See, Smell, and Know* (New York: Scribner, 2010).

[5]Martin Luther, "Table Talk," May 18, 1532, *Luther's Works* 54 (Philadelphia: Fortress Press, 1967), 37, 38.

[6]John Homans, quoted in Maria Povava, "The Enviable Dimwittedness of Dogs," *Atlantic*, December 7, 2012, www.theatlantic.com/health/archive /2012/12/the-enviable-dimwittedness-of-a-dog/266041.

[7]Along with Martin Luther and C. S. Lewis, I believe that dogs (and other animals) will have a part in the new heaven and the new earth, but I will not make that case here.

CHAPTER 16: MISS BECKY AND A WAY OF SPEAKING

[1]Larry Silver, "Executive Function Disorder, Explained!" *Additude*, accessed March 16, 2017, www.additudemag.com/adhd/article/7051.html.

CHAPTER 17: WORDS FAIL US

[1]These are collected in Edwin Newman, *Edwin Newman on Language: Strictly Speaking* and *A Civil Tongue* (New York: Galahad Books, 1992).

[2]On the significance of worship in the book of Revelation, see Robert Coleman, *Songs of Heaven* (Old Tappan, NJ: Revell, 1980).

CHAPTER 18: MY ESCAPE INTO MEANING

[1]The material in this chapter is adapted from Douglas Groothuis, "Bedeviled by My Wife's Dementia," *Christianity Today*, October 26, 2015, www .christianitytoday.com/ct/2015/november/bedeviled-by-my-wifes -dementia.html.

[2]W. Terrence Gordon, *Marshall McLuhan: Escape into Understanding* (Berkeley, CA: Gingko Press, 2003).

[3]Bruce Cockburn, "Broken Wheel," *Inner City Front*, 1981.

[4]J. R. R. Tolkien, "On Fairy Stories," in *Myth, Allegory, and Gospel*, ed. John Warwick Montgomery (Minneapolis: Bethany House, 1973).

[5]See Douglas Groothuis, "The Book, the Screen, and the Soul," in *The Soul in Cyberspace* (Grand Rapids: Baker, 1997).

[6]Marva Dawn, "Behold," in *Talking the Walk: Letting Christian Language Live Again* (Grand Rapids: Brazos, 2005).

[7]See Francis Schaeffer, *The God Who Is There*, 30th anniversary ed. (Downers Grove, IL: InterVarsity Press, 1998).

[8]See Peter Gay, *Modernism: The Lure of Heresy* (New York: W. W. Norton, 2010).

[9]See Kevin Whitehead, *Why Jazz?* (Oxford University Press, 2011); and Douglas Groothuis, "How to Listen to Jazz," *All About Jazz*, January 22, 2015, www.allaboutjazz.com/how-to-listen-to-jazz-by-douglas-groothuis.php.

[10]Richard Mouw makes a strong case that the new heaven and new earth will feature all that was good in all of human culture. I agree, but will not make that case here. See his *When the Kings Come Marching In* (Grand Rapids: Eerdmans, 1983).

INTERLUDE: BECKY AS MY STUDENT

[1]It was 1 Chronicles 12:32: "from Issachar, men who understood the times and knew what Israel should do—200 chiefs, with all their relatives under their command."

CHAPTER 19: HOW IS BECKY?

[1]See Danielle Steel, *His Bright Life: The Story of Nick Traina* (New York: Delta, 1998).

[2]Danielle Steel, "About Me," *Danielle Steel* (blog), accessed March 15, 2017, www.daniellesteel.net/about.htm.

APPENDIX

[1]The material in this appendix is adapted from Douglas Groothuis, "Suffering Well with Others," *The Constructive Curmudgeon* (blog), October 13, 2005, http://theconstructivecurmudgeon.blogspot.com/2005/10/suffering-well -with-others.html.

[2]Nicholas Wolterstorff, *Lament for a Son* (Grand Rapids: Eerdmans, 1987), 34.

[3]Christopher Hitchens, *Hitch-22* (New York: Twelve, 2006), 1.

[4]Judith Martin, *Miss Manners' Guide for the Turn of the Millennium* (New York: Fireside, 1989), 292.